'An inspiring celebration of the milestones and motivation of running's greatest stars, In The Running also lauds the everyday heroes at the back of the pack. Encyclopaedic and engaging, you'll delight in its many tales of courage, camaraderie and sheer craziness.'

Lisa Jackson, author of *Your Pace or Mine?*

'A fascinating look at the limits of human endurance – informative, inspiring, but above all entertaining.'

Kate Mosse, author and broadcaster

'For women, it's not just about running. It's about changing their lives. Phil Hewitt captures this in his compelling narrative of these astonishing women who have created this sport.'

Kathrine Switzer, pioneer of women's marathon running and leader of the 261 Fearless Movement

'What a marvellous idea for a book about the most fascinating characters in the history of distance running! No one is better fitted to tell their stories than Phil Hewitt, a brilliant wordsmith devoted to the sport.'

Peter Lovesey, novelist and athletics historian

C016258710

IN THE RUNNING

IN THE RUNNING

Summersdale Publishers Ltd
46 West Street
Chichester
West Sussex
PO19 1RP
UK

www.summersdale.com

Printed and bound by CPI Group (UK) Ltd, Croydon, CR0 4YY

ISBN: 978-1-84953-886-2

IN THE RUNNING

STORIES OF EXTRAORDINARY RUNNERS FROM AROUND THE WORLD

PHIL HEWITT

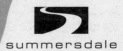

summersdale

About the Author

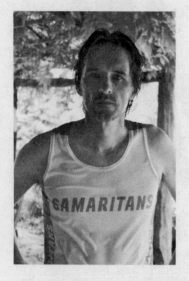

Phil Hewitt was brought up in Gosport, Hampshire, where he attended Bay House School. He later gained a first-class honours degree in modern languages and a doctorate in early twentieth-century French theatre from Oxford University. He joined the *Chichester Observer* in 1990 and became the newspaper's arts editor four years later. He is now also arts editor for all the Observer's sister papers across West Sussex, including the *West Sussex Gazette* and the *West Sussex County Times*.

Phil lives in Bishops Waltham, Hampshire, with his wife Fiona and children Adam and Laura. A keen runner, he has completed 30 marathons including London six times, Paris three times, plus New York, Berlin, Dublin, Rome, Mallorca, Amsterdam, Marrakech and Tokyo among others. Phil is also the author of *Keep on Running, Chichester Then and Now, Chichester Remembered, Gosport Then and Now, A Chichester Miscellany, A Portsmouth Miscellany* and *A Winchester Miscellany*. You can also follow him on Twitter at **@marathon_addict**.

CONTENTS

13   **INTRODUCTION**

15   **CHAPTER ONE: RUNNING FINDS ITS FEET**
Pheidippides (GR) – How it all began
Deerfoot (US) – The whooping warrior
Charles Rowell (GB) – The Cambridge Wonder
Dorando Pietri (IT) – Everyone's favourite loser
Arthur Newton (GB) – The father of long-distance running
Paavo Nurmi (FI) – The Flying Finn
Roger Bannister (GB) – Breaking the 4-minute mile

38   **CHAPTER TWO: TRULY INSPIRATIONAL**
Jane Tomlinson (GB) – An inspiration to millions
Hyvon Ngetich (KE) – A remarkable finish
Eddie Izzard (GB) – The comedian who ran his way
   into the nation's hearts
Terry Fox (CA) – The Marathon of Hope
Bruce Cleland (NZ) – The world's first charity runner
Jennifer Sheridan (US) – 'Be good, be strong'

56   **CHAPTER THREE: THE PIONEERS OF WOMEN'S
DISTANCE RUNNING**
Violet Piercy (GB) – A true pioneer of women's running
Dale Greig (GB) – Followed by an ambulance

Bobbi Gibb (GB) – Joining the men
Kathrine Switzer (US) – A pioneer of women's
   marathon running
Miki Gorman (US) – Conquering the doubts

73   CHAPTER FOUR: BECAUSE IT'S THERE
Dave McGillivray (US) – The race director who runs
   his years
Amy Hughes (GB) – 53 marathons in 53 days
Kim Allan (NZ) – Three and a half days without sleep
Achim Aretz (DE) – Putting your best foot backwards!
Fiona Oakes (GB) – The meat-free athlete
Jon Sutherland (US) – The greatest, unbroken
   running streak
Rick Worley (US) – Something for the weekend!
David and Linda Major (GB) – A marathon couple
Jen Correa (US) – Running back to normality

**96   CHAPTER FIVE: THE LEGENDS OF MEN'S
DISTANCE RUNNING**
Emil Zátopek (CZ) – A unique triple Olympic win
Jim Peters (GB)– Disaster after run of
   record-breaking marathons
Kip Keino (KE) – Paving the way
Steve Prefontaine (US) – The Muhammad
   Ali of distance running
Chris Brasher (GB) – The man who created the
   London Marathon
Haile Gebrselassie (ET) – World records tumble
Paul Tergat (KE) – No more Mr Silver

119 **CHAPTER SIX: DEFEATING THE TERRORISTS**

Theresa Giammona (US) – Honouring a beloved husband

Kevin Parks (US) – Building a network of support

Brian Kelley (US) – The running world unites

Juli Windsor (US) – Overcoming disability and terrorist attack

Lynn Crisci (US) – Survivor turned marathon runner

George Salines (FR)– The man who kept running

136 **CHAPTER SEVEN: CONQUERING DISABILITY**

David Kuhn (US) – The blind runner running to beat cystic fibrosis

Team Hoyt (US) – More than a thousand races together

The Schneider twins (US) – Running with autism

Claire Lomas (GB) – 'The making of me'

Maickel Melamed (VE)– A glorious finish against all the odds

Phil Packer (GB)– The London Marathon in 14 days

151 **CHAPTER EIGHT: THE 80s GREATS OF WOMEN'S DISTANCE RUNNING**

Grete Waitz (NO) – Nine-time New York City champion

Ingrid Kristiansen (NO) – The other half of a great rivalry

Rosa Mota (PT) – Olympic dreams

Joan Benoit Samuelson (US) – A giant among runners

164 **CHAPTER NINE: WHEN THE MIND IS WILLING**

Kim Stemple (US) – With strength to share

Patrick Finney (US) – The first runner with MS to complete a marathon in every US state

Elizabeth Maiuolo (AR) – 'Getting my heart back to perfect shape'

Michael LaForgia (US) – Overcoming double amputation

Don Wright (US) – The great survivor

Mark McGirr (US) – Running back from the dead

176 CHAPTER TEN: PUSHING THE LIMITS OF HUMAN ENDURANCE

Ted Jackson (GB) – Seven in seven on seven for MS

Angela Tortorice (US) – The women's record for the most marathons in a year

Dean Karnazes (US) – The man who can run forever

Stefaan Engels (BE) – A year in marathons

Rob Young (GB) – The most marathons in a year

Kevin Carr (GB) – The fastest man around the world

Paul Staso (US) – Keeping a promise to the children

Cliff Young (AU) – The man who gave us the Young Shuffle

Marathon Maniac Larry (US) – Record after record

Istvan Sipos (HU) – Running to infinity

JC Santa Teresa (US) – The most successive ultramarathons

202 CHAPTER ELEVEN: IN THE TOUGHEST PLACES

Mauro Prosperi (IT) – Drinking bats' blood to survive

Dave Heeley (GB) – Running blind through the desert

Engle, Zahab and Lin (US, CA, TW) – 4,000 miles across the Sahara

Scott Jurek (US) – A modern Pheidippides
Pat Farmer (AU) – 'A burning desire to get back
   to basics'
Scott and Rhys Jenkins (GB) – The hottest place on earth
Sir Ranulph Fiennes (GB) – 'The world's greatest
   living explorer'
Nicholas Bourne (GB) – The length of Africa, twice
Malcolm Attard (GB) – On top of the world

228   **CHAPTER TWELVE: AGE SHALL NOT WEARY...**
Fauja Singh (GB) – Probably the world's oldest
   marathon runner
Bob Dolphin (US) – 500 marathons and counting
Joy Johnson (US) – A marathoner to the end
Louise Rossetti (US) – Overcoming personal tragedy
Sister Madonna Buder (US) – The Iron Nun
Sab Koide (US) – Cab fare not needed
Gladys Burrill and Harriette Thompson (US) –
   The world's oldest female marathoners

245   **CHAPTER THIRTEEN: THE MODERN GREATS**
Catherine Ndereba (KE) – Catherine the Great
Tegla Loroupe (KE) – Championing peace
   and social change
Paula Radcliffe (GB) – Still no one else is coming close
Mary Keitany (KE) – The power of motherhood
Geoffrey Mutai (KE) – The world record that wasn't
Kenenisa Bekele (ET) – A stunning marathon debut
Sammy Wanjiru (KE) – A tragic loss to marathon running
Dennis Kimetto (KE) – Chasing the 2-hour marathon
Mo Farah (GB) – 'It's great to make history'

278 **CHAPTER FOURTEEN: THE MOST EXTRAORDINARY RUN OF ALL**
Tim Peake (GB) – Out of this world!

282 **REFERENCES**

INTRODUCTION

Why do we run? It's the age-old question — the question to which there are as many answers as there are runners. The elite run to be the best in the world; many millions run simply to improve their times; others run to be better versions of themselves. Some run to challenge who they are, to inspire others or to champion their cause; others run to say no to illness and improve their health.

For others still, running is a way to say yes to humanity, to force social change, to bring about integration and to break down prejudice; others run to stick two fingers up to petty officialdom and silly regulations; as we saw at the Paris Marathon in 2016 and at Boston in 2014, there are plenty of runners who run to shout a deafening no to those who spread terror.

And then there are the runners who run to defy the elements, through scorching heat and freezing cold; they run to conquer new territories, to take mind and body to places they have never been and will never go again; others run to raise millions for charity, and they run through hope and despair.

You will find all these stories and more in this book: tales of the runners who never feel more alive than when they are running; of ambitions fulfilled and shattered; of feats that surpass anything that has ever gone before; of runners who have changed their world and ours for the better; of runners who have gone to the brink and back and have left their mark.

All of life is here – a celebration of the runners for whom life is running and running is life.

Linking them all is the fact that for runners everywhere, running is essentially freedom. For the very best, it's the freedom to *be* the very best; for the rest of us, it's all about reclaiming something equally precious: our right to be ourselves away from all the pressures of modern-day living.

That was certainly the case with me. Running is the perfect antidote to work and the best possible way to appreciate all the pleasures of home life. It's been about rebalancing.

But it has also been about touching greatness. I still pinch myself to think that I was running in the same London Marathon in which Paula Radcliffe set the fastest ever time for a woman marathoner in 2003 and that I also ran (as a total also-ran) in the same Berlin Marathon in which Haile Gebrselassie broke his own record in 2008 to set a new men's record. 'You were my tailwind and are all record-breaking runners, too!' he told the rest of us. I love that thought. We were privileged to be there.

In 2012, I wrote a book called *Keep on Running*, an attempt to explain to myself why I run. I'm not sure I ever did come up with an answer. In many ways, this is a companion volume, an attempt to find out why *other* people run. Here you will find the stories of a hundred runners who have gone the course.

Inevitably, this is a very personal selection of stories: tales that appeal to me and that I hope will appeal to you. We each champion different champions, and therein lies much of the fun.

So let's jump in. And as I said in *Keep on Running*, I hope you will still be with me at the finishing line.

CHAPTER ONE
RUNNING FINDS ITS FEET

Pheidippides – How it all began

*'Their imagination is stirred by the idea of
being a modern Pheidippides, running in
the footsteps of the ancient messenger.'*

Although his name is not well known today, the race he ran
certainly is. But did it really happen in the way that legend has
passed it down to us? Did Pheidippides really run a marathon
to announce that Athenian democracy had been saved and then
promptly drop down dead?

No one knows, and no one can ever know. But the story is
irresistible. It would be awful to think it all started prosaically at
a committee meeting somewhere. You want the opening chapter
in the story of mankind's love affair with long-distance running
to be dramatic, and Pheidippides' tale is certainly that – tragic yet
glorious, defeated yet undefeated, sad but heroic.

It seems entirely appropriate and appropriately epic as the starting point for the long-distance feats which millions of us have pursued ever since. We love distance running *but* it hurts. We love it *because* it hurts. We love it because it takes us to the extremes – though ideally not the one Pheidippides experienced.

The modern Athens marathon – and arguably all marathons everywhere – commemorate Pheidippides' moment of fame. He ran around 26 miles from a battlefield at the site of the town of Marathon to Athens in 490 BC to bring news of a Greek victory over the Persians. Legend has it that the poor chap's final words were '*Niki!*' ('Victory') or '*Nenikikamen!*' ('Rejoice we conquer', that is 'We have won'). Run a marathon and chances are you will know how he felt.

The August heat would have been a factor in his subsequent demise. But also significant is the fact that apparently he had already been putting in the miles. Athens needed the help of the Spartans for their stand against the Persians at Marathon, and Pheidippides' first run, lasting some 36 hours, had been 140 miles (some say 147) to Sparta… and back.

It seems the Spartans were willing to help, but, in accordance with their religious laws, they wouldn't fight until full moon. Or maybe they just didn't want to. Either way, any help would be too late. By profession and practice a trained runner, it was Pheidippides' sorry task to run back with the bad news. Having delivered it, he then fought in the unlikely victory that followed, after which he promptly embarked on his more famous run, off to Athens to announce the victory – a total of more than 300 miles in just one week.

Whether the same runner who had been to Sparta and back really carried out this third run is questionable. Historians will continue to argue it either way, just as they will continue to ponder why he didn't travel by horse and whether he really did die at the end of it – speculations which ought to be dismissed for the party-pooping fact that they try to stand in the way of a good story, the birth of our modern marathon.

The first modern Olympic games were held in 1896 in Greece, and in the marathon, it was Pheidippides that the games honoured with a 40,000-metre (24.85-mile) run from Marathon Bridge to the Olympic stadium in Athens – a race which assumed huge importance for the home crowd. The marathon has become traditionally the final event in the Olympics, and on 10 April 1896, Greece was still waiting for its first medal. With its historical significance, the marathon was the race the nation wanted to win more than any other. Greek postal worker (or maybe shepherd, depending on whom you believe) Spiridon Louis (1873–1940) was the man they pinned their hopes on. Some say he prepared for the race by praying for two days and fasting for one. Some accounts – disputed elsewhere – even suggest he had a glass of wine en route. He let no one down, coming home in a time of 2 hours 58 minutes 50 seconds.

It was a victory that made him a hero of the modern Olympic movement. He soon spawned his own mythology. Some accounts say his prize was free meals for a year, a field, a horse and cart and free shoe polishing for life. More certain is the fact that it was Louis who was chosen to offer Adolf Hitler an olive branch at the start of the 1936 Olympic Games in Berlin. Some you win. Some you lose…

At the 1908 Olympic Games in London, the marathon distance was changed to 26.2 miles to cover the ground from Windsor Castle to White City Stadium, with a finish in front of the royal family's viewing box. It was confirmed as the standard marathon distance at the 1924 Olympics in Paris.

Pheidippides' story also lives on in the modern Spartathlon, a historic ultradistance footrace that takes place in Greece every September. The race was conceived when John Foden, a British RAF wing commander and a student of ancient Greek history, paused in his reading of Herodotus and wondered if modern man could cover the distance from Athens to Sparta, 250 km, within 36 hours, as Pheidippides was said to have done. Foden and four colleagues from the RAF put themselves to the test in 1982 and succeeded. A new race was born.

Deerfoot – The whooping warrior

*'His appearance caused a great rush
to obtain a peek at him.'*

Scantily clad and blisteringly fast, Deerfoot was always going to make an impact, particularly in Victorian London. No one had ever seen anyone quite like him before.

Born in around 1830 on the Cattaraugus Reservation in Upstate New York, Lewis Bennett, Hut-goh-so-do-neh in his native tongue and known in running circles as Deerfoot, was a Seneca Indian and one of the leading runners of the nineteenth century. The story goes that as a youngster he outpaced a horse for some 30 or 40 miles before the horse eventually died of exhaustion.

Deerfoot first came to public attention in 1856 when he won a 5-mile race at Fredonia, New York in 25 minutes, an outstanding time for the period and still a pretty good one even now. As a result, America's long-distance champion John Grindell travelled to New York to challenge him – and lost.

Alert to Bennett's feats, George Martin, a British promoter, renamed him Deerfoot and set out to make him a star, bringing him to England in 1861 on a 20-month running tour which saw him beat nearly all the best long-distance runners in the world. At nearly 183 cm (6 feet) tall, running bare chested at first and with his dark complexion, he cut the most striking of figures. He declined to wear running spikes, preferring to run in moccasins, and for his publicity appearances, he wore a wolfskin blanket, a headband and an eagle feather. Before his first race, the *London Sporting News* tried to convey the excitement he caused:

> *His appearance caused a great rush to obtain a peek at him as he stalked in stately manner, with his wolf skin wrapped around him, looking the very model of one of Fenimore Cooper's Mohicans or Pawnees.*

Adding to the mystique was the fact that he never said a word. Martin had told people he didn't speak English. Part also of the persona were the tactics he adopted, storming past an opponent and then slowing down again. Once they had caught him, he would race ahead again. He ran an inconsistent pace, repeatedly surging. He also liked to treat his fans to warrior whoops, in order to remind them of his Native American origins.

And it worked. Victory after victory followed as Deerfoot travelled around England for the rest of the year, running 15 more races in 13 weeks and winning all but one. He was mystery and entertainer rolled into one. With his long, powerful strides, he wasn't a graceful runner, but he was certainly a striking one, swinging his body from side to side and rolling his head as he passed through.

Inevitably he attracted attention. In November 1861, the Prince of Wales invited him to run in a 6-mile race in Cambridge. Deerfoot won. The Prince of Wales duly presented him with a watch and two banknotes. He even dined with the future Edward VII in Trinity College.

The public was entranced. Martin responded with plans for a travelling Deerfoot Circus, aimed at maximising profits, with Deerfoot available to all comers. However, there was controversy early in 1862. Allegations persisted that Deerfoot's exhibition races were fixed. In the public backlash, Martin resolved that the best way to restore lost credibility was to set world records, something Deerfoot had previously taken no interest in. However, Deerfoot duly delivered. On 2 November 1862, in a 1-hour race at Brompton, he set the new standard with a record-breaking 11 miles 720 yards – a record he bettered when he ran 11 miles 790 yards on 12 January 1863 at Hackney Wick. In all, he went on to set new 10-, 11- and 12-mile records.

However, his performances fell away soon afterwards, and he returned to the States where he continued to compete at a lower level until 1870. On his death in the 1890s, on the Cattaraugus Reservation where he had been born, the *New York Times* noted, 'Deerfoot, the Fleet, is no more.' He is buried in Forest Lawn Cemetery, Buffalo, New York.

Charles Rowell – The Cambridge Wonder

'In his prime undoubtedly the finest long distance runner the world has ever seen.'
OTTAWA CITIZEN

They were called pedestrians, but there was nothing remotely pedestrian about their feats. As so-called 'pedestrian mania' gripped the sporting world in the late 1870s, a new generation of walking and running stars was emerging. Crowds gathered in their thousands at tracks around the world to watch men walking and running through sawdust for up to six days and nights at a time, with the promise of wealth beyond their dreams as their reward.

Pedestrianism, a form of competitive walking which eventually gave birth to the modern sport of race walking, had emerged in England as far back as 1765, but it reached its height in a golden decade, 1875–1885. One of the greats of the era was Charles Rowell (1852–1909), the Cambridge Wonder, the boatman who turned record breaker.

Edward Payson Weston was perhaps the man who did most to promote the popularity of pedestrianism in the nineteenth century. In 1861, he walked from Boston to Washington, DC; in 1867, he walked 1,226 miles from Portland, Maine to Chicago. A craze was gathering pace. The last quarter of the nineteenth century in the United States saw a proliferation of runs based on time (24, 48 or 72 hours or six days) or distance (25, 50 or 100 miles).

Weston himself pioneered the six-day race; British nobleman Sir John Astley took it to the next level when he sponsored five international races for hefty prize money plus a championship gold and silver belt, which bore the legend 'Long-distance Champion of the World'.

Weston and Astley were both to prove key figures in Rowell's life. An admirer of Weston, Rowell had been working in his youth in Foster's boatyard in Cambridge until his hero's exploits prompted him to turn pedestrian as well. In his early running days, Rowell would think nothing of running 56 miles to London to consult with Astley on business, only to run back the next day, generally taking 6 hours. A future champion was taking his first strides.

Rousing fierce nationalistic pride and attracting thousands of spectators on two separate continents, Astley's six-day and six-night marathon races were spread over an 18-month period either side of the Atlantic, and dubbed 'go-as-you-please' matches. Under intense scrutiny of all kinds, contestants could walk or run, and they could rest whenever they wanted – though they rarely rested more than a few hours out of every 24. All they had to do was keep to the rules. Unsurprisingly, they were huge magnets for the bookies.

The first of the Astley Belt races took place in London's Agricultural Hall starting on 18 March 1878 and was won by the Irish-born American champion Daniel O'Leary, who covered 520 miles in 139 hours; the second race, in New York's Madison Square Garden later that year, again saw O'Leary victorious. However, in the third, again at Madison Square Garden, starting on 10 March 1879, a new hero emerged: the Englishman Charles Rowell. Previously a sprinter at 20–50-mile races, it was the first time he had attempted a six-day 'go-as-you-please' grind, but the Cambridge Wonder took the honours, running 500 miles to win $20,000, the equivalent of just over $1 million today.

Competition was fierce. Weston, the supreme showman of the pedestrian world, was waiting, and formally challenged Rowell to the next race, the fourth match back at London's Agricultural Hall on 16 June 1879. After stepping on a nail, Rowell had to sit it out, but he was fit again that autumn and recaptured the belt in the fifth and final Astley Belt contest, which began on 22 September

1879. Despite suffering 'a fit of convulsions' not long before the race, he secured $30,000 for his week's work, notching up 530 miles, 15 ahead of second place.

Rowell managed 550 miles the following year, though in 1884, fellow Englishman George Littlewood took the record with a remarkable 623.75 miles in 139 hours 59 minutes, still a record today. However, by then Rowell had managed to acquire a new record of his own, running 300 miles indoors in 58:17:06 (27 February–1 March 1882), a feat which has yet to be beaten, either outdoors or in. He also ran 89 miles in 12 hours and 150 miles in 23 hours.

Such was his fame and indeed his reputation that, on one occasion, backers of his opponents drugged his food. Rowell was the man to beat, by fair means or foul.

With his repeated success, Rowell did indeed secure the promised untold riches, but his later years were sad ones. His obituary in the *New Zealand Herald* on 16 October 1909 carried the headline 'Made £70,000, but ended his life in poverty'. It noted:

> *Charles Rowell, in his best days the finest long distance runner in the world, died recently at Cambridge, after a long illness. He had fallen on evil days, and died practically destitute.*

The *Ottawa Citizen*, in its obituary on the same date, also labelled him the finest, estimating he acquired a fortune of $100,000 'only to lose it in speculation on the turf' – a miserable end for a true great.

Dorando Pietri – Everyone's favourite loser

*'The Italian's great performance can never
be effaced from our record of sport, be the
decision of the judges what it may.'*
ARTHUR CONAN DOYLE

Rarely can the achievement have seemed greater. Rarely can the judgement of the authorities have seemed harsher. Epic fail is a beloved expression these days. It might have been invented for Dorando Pietri, the runner who won and lost the 1908 Olympic marathon. As the *New York Times* put it:

> *It would be no exaggeration to say that the finish of the marathon at the 1908 Olympics in London was the most thrilling athletic event that has occurred since that marathon race in ancient Greece, where the victor fell at the goal and, with a wave of triumph, died.*

Pietri, a confectioner from Carpi, Italy, was clearly disorientated as he staggered into the Olympic stadium at Shepherd's Bush where a crowd of 100,000 was roaring him on. Some people say there were a million more outside. But it wasn't to be Pietri's day. He wobbled and fell. He then staggered back to his feet, only to fall again. Doctors and officials surrounded him but did him no favours. Pietri's chance, however slim, disappeared the moment the day's chief medical officer Michael Bulger went to his aid. Jack Andrew, the clerk of the course, tried in vain to hold Bulger back.

Years later Andrew's daughter discovered her father's account of the race:

> As Dorando reached the track he staggered and after a few yards fell. I kept would-be helpers at bay, but Dr Bulger went to his assistance. I warned him that this would entail disqualification, but he replied that although I was in charge of the race, I must obey him. Each time Dorando fell I had to hold his legs while the doctor massaged him to keep his heart beating.

The crowd begged, and the doctors and officials gave way: they dragged the unconscious runner over the finishing line. The applause was deafening, but not as deafening as the disapproval of the race authorities who inevitably and understandably disqualified him. Their argument was irrefutable: Pietri had been helped over the line. The American John Joseph Hayes won instead. *Sport Illustrato* described the ruling as 'draconian and pitiless'. Sir Arthur Conan Doyle also caught the flavour of Pietri's finish: 'It is horrible, yet fascinating, this struggle between a set purpose and an utterly exhausted frame.'

Queen Alexandra didn't have to play it by the rules, however. Pietri hovered near death for several hours after the race. When he recovered, Queen Alexandra presented him with an enormous gold cup. The authorities applied the letter of the law. The queen read the mood of the nation.

The decision, the public response and the royal accolade all made a hero of Pietri – and perhaps also of running. It's perfectly possible to argue that his misfortune was a major factor in the surge of popularity marathon running subsequently enjoyed. Pietri became an international celebrity on the back of his London misery. Irving Berlin dedicated a song to him entitled 'Dorando', and invitations flowed in for exhibition races in the United States, including a rematch against Hayes in New York's Madison Square Garden on 25 November 1908. Pietri duly won. He enjoyed repeated success on his tour of America and during his three years of professional running.

Pietri died in 1942, aged 56. On the centenary of his London fall, his home town remembered him. A statue was unveiled in Carpi, called Dorando the Winner.

For the record Pietri's time was 2 hours 54 minutes 46 seconds. The event was the first marathon to be run at the new distance of 26 miles 385 yards (42.2 km), the distance which has since become standard.

Arthur Newton – The father of long-distance running

'There has departed also the greatest
gentleman of them all.'
THE TIMES

If they want a good day, runners in South Africa's celebrated Comrades Marathon must honour Arthur at the halfway mark at Drummond. Race organisers remind runners that when they run past the Wall of Honour – also known as Arthur's Seat – they should pay tribute. Tradition dictates that they place flowers at the spot, take off their hats, bow and say 'Good morning, sir' – a rather quaint tradition that also acknowledges one of the race's greats.

The 89-km (55.3-mile) Comrades Marathon is acknowledged as one of the world's greatest ultramarathons, a South African institution notorious for the body-sapping challenge it poses and for the camaraderie it fosters among its thousands of participants. Run between the capital of the KwaZulu-Natal province, Pietermaritzburg, and the coastal city of Durban, the race alternates annually between the 'up run' from Durban and the 'down run' from Pietermaritzburg.

And in its early years, it was undoubtedly Arthur's race. Comrades Marathon Association chairman Peter Proctor is among the many to acknowledge five-time winner Arthur Newton's part in its history:

> *It is rumoured that in the good old days Arthur took a rest and had a sandwich and something to drink at the seat. It is now a tradition of Comrades Marathon that all runners run past that seat and take off their hats just to greet Arthur and it's also rumoured that if runners do not take off their hats, they will not have a nice race from there on, but of course that might just be all a rumour...*

The race, first run in 1921, was the idea of First World War veteran Vic Clapham who wanted to commemorate the South African soldiers who had been killed in the conflict. Clapham had himself endured a 2,700-km (1,677-mile) route march through German East Africa. Inevitably, he wanted his race to be a recognition of man's endurance or, as the race literature says, a celebration of 'mankind's spirit over adversity'.

Arthur Francis Hamilton Newton (1883–1959) was born in Weston-super-Mare in the UK. He initially went to South Africa in 1901 to join his brother. He settled in Durban and became a teacher, before deciding in 1909 to settle permanently in South Africa, acquiring a farm in Natal two years later. During the First World War, Newton served as a trooper in the Natal Light Horse and also as a dispatch rider. However, while he was fighting, his farm was suffering. African workers burnt much of his pasture land, and machinery was destroyed. Newton, a quiet, self-effacing man, blamed the union government and demanded compensation. When he didn't get it, he determined to take his fight to the next level, and for that he realised he needed publicity. Newton turned to running to highlight his grievance.

As he later said:

> *Genuine amateur athletics were about as wholesome as anything on this earth; any man who made a really notable name at such would always be given a hearing by the public.*

And this was the reason he entered the Comrades Marathon. He had a problem, however. He couldn't run 2 miles without stopping. His response was to evolve his own regime of fitness training. It worked. In 1922, with his characteristic swing-trot, he launched into the first of a remarkable series of Comrades victories. His debut success, finishing in 8 hours 40 minutes, startled everyone, not least Newton himself.

> *It came as a surprise to myself. I rather thought I could run into*

*third or fourth place, but certainly I did not
expect to win, and still less to cover the course
in under 9 hours 15 minutes.*

The following year, surprise turned to astonishment. As the race
official history notes:

> *Newton had come home in the
> unbelievable time of 6 hours and
> 56 minutes, having thus broken
> the 7-hour barrier. There can be no doubt,
> the Comrades Marathon was never the same
> again after such an epic run.*

The following year, 1924, Newton won again, this time in the
slightly slower time of 6 hours 58 minutes – despite collapsing
after taking a fizzy drink. That same year, he had gone back to
England where he broke the London-to-Brighton record by
more than an hour, finishing in a time of 5:53:43. His finest year,
however, came in 1925 when he secured his fourth Comrades
victory, at the age of 42. At the peak of his fitness, he was home
in 6 hours 24 minutes, improving a massive 31 minutes on his
previous best. Newton secured his fifth and final Comrades win in
1927, finishing in 6:40:56.

But still no compensation was forthcoming. In the end, Newton
resolved to move to Rhodesia to be in a 'British country', but
with no money, he was forced to set out on his 770-mile journey
on foot, walking at night out of sheer embarrassment at his
poverty. Eventually, he was lent a bicycle. Once in Rhodesia, he
continued to run, setting new records for 60 and 100 miles on
roads. In January 1928, back in England, Newton broke the 100-

mile record between Bath and London. Turning professional, he enjoyed continued success.

Long after his own running ceased, he remained an avid supporter and student of the sport, writing a series of influential books on the subject. On his death, in Middlesex, on 7 September 1959, he was acknowledged as the father of modern long-distance running.

Paavo Nurmi – The Flying Finn

'Mind is everything. Muscle – pieces of rubber.
All that I am, I am because of my mind.'

You would expect superstars to live in a different zone to mere mortals. The Flying Finn Paavo Nurmi (1897–1973) certainly did. One of the most successful male athletes in Olympic history and one of only four athletes to win nine Olympic gold medals, he was also one of his sport's great enigmas, a seemingly unknowable man who kept his mystery intact to the end. 'All that I am, I am because of my mind,' he famously said; and into that mind, he let no one.

Nurmi made his Olympic debut at the 1920 Antwerp Games, winning gold medals in the 10,000 m and the cross-country individual and team events. He also claimed silver in the 5,000 m. In fact, he was only warming up. At the 1924 Paris Games he made history, becoming the first athlete ever to win five gold medals at a single Olympics. In just four days, Nurmi won successively the 1,500 m, the 5,000 m, the two cross-country events and the 3,000 m team event. In two of those events, the 1,500 m and 5,000 m runs, he set two Olympic records in little more than an hour.

The world hadn't seen anything like this before, and his influence on the track world was immense. Some would argue we haven't seen his like since. Nurmi took his chosen sport to a higher level and made it the focus of global attention.

On 23 August 1923, in Stockholm, Nurmi set a mile record, running each of the first three quarters (440 yards) in exactly 63 seconds and then the final quarter in 61.4 seconds. His record-breaking 4 minutes 10.4 seconds remained the fastest mile ever for the next eight years. Arguably it was one of his greatest achievements. In all, he set 22 world records across a range of distances.

The world could see his brilliance. However, the world struggled to understand it. Nurmi was the winner who never smiled. Clearly popularity was never on his agenda. Observers noted that he seemed to run without pleasure even as he continued to plunder the records. The *Guardian* pondered his mystery in 1925:

> *What is there about this phlegmatic Finn that makes him the superior of every other athlete who has ever pulled on a spiked shoe? He is slight, fair-haired, sometimes moody, and always temperamental. He has magnificent thighs and nicely-rounded calves, but there is nothing about him that suggests the super-man the stop-watches have proved him to be.*

Gabriel Hanot, writing in *Le Miroir des Sports*, was among those who took issue with the way the 27-year-old Nurmi came across publicly. Hanot also posed a question which was to become one of the key talking points of Nurmi's career. Was Nurmi truly an amateur?

> *Paavo Nurmi lives beyond humanity. He is ever more serious, reserved,*

concentrated, pessimistic, fanatic. There is such coldness in him and his self-control is so great that never for a moment does he show his feelings [...] What is Paavo Nurmi's mentality? Why does he seem to lack human qualities? Is he a slave of sport, of training, of records, in such degree that he sacrifices his body and soul with no thought, regard or free moment spared for the outside world?

Sadly, Nurmi's career ended in controversy. At the 1928 Amsterdam Olympics, Nurmi won the 10,000 m and silver medals in the 5,000 m and the steeplechase. His main-attraction status was his undoing, however. The sport's governing body, the International Association of Athletics Federations (IAAF), declared him to be a professional, which meant he missed out on the 1932 Olympic Games in Los Angeles and a possible tenth gold medal. There were furious protests in Helsinki, and even his fellow competitors supported him. Finland fought the ban as hard as it could. Nurmi even travelled with the team to America, but two days before the Games began, Nurmi had to concede that the ban was not going to be lifted. Argument continued to rage. Significantly, even after his Olympic dreams were shattered, Nurmi refused to turn professional. He continued to run as an amateur until his retirement from the sport in 1934.

Paavo Nurmi's greatest achievements

Event	Olympic Games	Medal
Men's 5,000 m	1920 Antwerp	Silver

Men's 10,000 m	1920 Antwerp	Gold
Men's cross-country, individual	1920 Antwerp	Gold
Men's cross-country, team	1920 Antwerp	Gold
Men's 1,500 m	1924 Paris	Gold
Men's 5,000 m	1924 Paris	Gold
Men's 3,000 m, team	1924 Paris	Gold
Men's cross-country, individual	1924 Paris	Gold
Men's cross-country, team	1924 Paris	Gold
Men's 5,000 m	1928 Amsterdam	Silver
Men's 10,000 m	1928 Amsterdam	Gold
Men's 3,000 m steeplechase	1928 Amsterdam	Silver

Roger Bannister – Breaking the 4-minute mile

*'I found longer races boring.
I found the mile just perfect.'*

The shoes Sir Roger Bannister wore to break the 4-minute mile were expected to fetch £50,000 when they came up for auction in September 2015. Snapped up by an anonymous buyer, they fetched £266,500 – a clear indication of just how much the young doctor's 'miracle mile' still resonates in our history.

Bannister's record has been broken no fewer than 18 times in the 62 years since he set it. In fact, it was first broken within a matter of weeks. But it still stands today as one of the great landmark moments in running history. At the time, the *Daily Telegraph* called it 'sport's greatest goal'. But as Bannister said himself: 'The man who can drive himself further once the effort gets painful is the man who will win.'

Bannister (*b.* 1929) had been predicted to win gold at the Olympic Games in Helsinki in 1952. He came fourth. Two years later, the expectation was that the 25-year-old medical student would run the 'miracle mile' at the Iffley Road Track in Oxford. Once president of the Oxford club, Bannister would be running for the Amateur Athletic Association against his old university during their annual match on 6 May 1954.

The pressure was on. Bannister prepared for the race the previous week at Paddington Green in London in high winds, but on the day he'd been waiting for, a 15-mph crosswind with gusts of up to 25 mph left Bannister wondering whether he should call the attempt off. Suddenly it seemed impossible. Bannister calculated with the wind he would lose a second a lap over the four laps, which meant he would have to run effectively 3 minutes 56 seconds to set the record – and he doubted he could do it. But after his morning house rounds at Paddington Hospital, he caught the train to Oxford anyway. As luck would have it, he bumped into his coach, Franz Stampfl, who told him he would never forgive himself if he didn't try.

And so he did.

Watched by about 3,000 spectators, Bannister set out, aided by two pacemakers, Chris Brasher and Chris Chataway, respectively the future founder of the London Marathon and a future Conservative MP. Everything came together, and Bannister sprinted over the line into the arms of his friend Rev Nicholas Stacey to record a time of 3 minutes 59.4 seconds. When the record was confirmed, so the BBC reported, pandemonium broke out.

Many athletes will tell you today there is a tendency – particularly in a metric world – to neglect the mile as one of the sport's most challenging distances, a distance which offers a true marker of greatness. Roger Bannister made it, briefly at least, the distance everyone was talking about.

Bannister's record lasted for 46 days, broken by John Landy, of Australia, when he ran a time of 3 minutes 58 seconds on 21 June 1954. Later that year, Bannister retired from running to pursue his medical studies full-time. He went on to become a consultant neurologist and was knighted in 1975.

Looking back on his achievement as its sixtieth anniversary approached, Bannister, in an interview in the *Daily Telegraph*, put his achievement in the wider context of growing post-war British optimism, the start of the new Elizabethan era: rationing was just ending, Everest had been conquered, a young queen was on the throne.

> Could Britain still make it in the post-war world? It seemed to be an emergence of some new kind of desire to excel and try to tackle physical barriers. We did have something which is not so fashionable now, a kind of patriotism.

Anyone who remembers it will remember he gave the whole country a boost in 3 minutes 59.4 seconds that changed running history.

Progress towards the fastest mile since 1940

Name	Location	Date	Time
Gunder Hägg	Sweden	1 July 1942	4:06.2
Arne Andersson	Sweden	10 July 1942	4:06.2
Gunder Hägg	Sweden	4 September 1942	4:04.6
Arne Andersson	Sweden	1 July 1943	4:02.6
Arne Andersson	Sweden	18 July 1944	4:01.6
Gunder Hägg	Sweden	17 July 1945	4:01.4
Roger Bannister	United Kingdom	6 May 1954	3:59.4
John Landy	Australia	21 June 1954	3:58.0
Derek Ibbotson	United Kingdom	19 July 1957	3:57.2
Herb Elliott	Australia	6 August 1958	3:54.5

Peter Snell	New Zealand	27 January 1962	3:54.4
Peter Snell	New Zealand	17 November 1964	3:54.1
Michel Jazy	France	9 June 1965	3:53.6
Jim Ryun	United States	17 July 1966	3:51.3
Jim Ryun	United States	23 June 1967	3:51.1
Filbert Bayi	Tanzania	17 May 1975	3:51.0
John Walker	New Zealand	12 August 1975	3:49.4
Sebastian Coe	United Kingdom	17 July 1979	3:48.95
Steve Ovett	United Kingdom	1 July 1980	3:48.8
Sebastian Coe	United Kingdom	19 August 1981	3:48.53
Steve Ovett	United Kingdom	26 August 1981	3:48.40
Sebastian Coe	United Kingdom	28 August 1981	3:47.33
Steve Cram	United Kingdom	27 July 1985	3:46.32
Noureddine Morceli	Algeria	5 September 1993	3:44.39
Hicham El Guerrouj	Morocco	7 July 1999	3:43.13

CHAPTER TWO
TRULY INSPIRATIONAL

Jane Tomlinson – An inspiration to millions

*'We all want to pass on
a bit of ourselves.'*

The London Marathon always throws up dozens of inspirational stories; few have been more inspirational than that of Jane Tomlinson, the plain-talking, strong-willed Yorkshire woman who captured attention and drew admiration worldwide with her seven-year refusal to give in to cancer.

Tomlinson, a radiographer and mother of three from Leeds, defied the disease through a string of remarkable achievements that still resonate today, inspiring thousands of people with memories of the cheerful courage which became her trademark. Tomlinson saw herself as a mum simply trying to make the most of a life she knew would end prematurely. She finished every challenge with a smile.

> *When I was first told I was going to die, my son was only three, and I could not bear the idea that he would not remember me. We all want to pass on a bit of ourselves into our children's lives, something that they can hold on to, I suppose. So I feel I have been blessed in that now he'll know a bit about who I was. At 36, I felt very much that I was too young to die, that I hadn't done enough, now at 40 I feel I have done more than a lot of people do in a lifetime. So if it's my time this year, I would say, 'Thank you, God, for what you gave me.' These precious four years. I mean how many other Yorkshire lasses do you know that can say they have cycled to Monte Carlo this afternoon?*

Tomlinson was 36 in August 2000 when she and her family were given the devastating news that she had terminal breast cancer. She was given six months to live. Her response was to set herself a string of challenges, which she fulfilled through her Jane Tomlinson Appeal, raising vast sums for research to help others.

The 2002 London Marathon was the beginning of Jane's fundraising and endurance feats. She confessed that she hadn't been particularly sporty beforehand, but training quickly became an important part of her life. Jane finished her first London Marathon in 4 hours 53 minutes and went on to complete a further two London Marathons. In 2003, Jane became the first person to run a marathon while receiving chemotherapy.

Many believed that her feats ought to have been impossible for someone suffering from cancer and undergoing chemotherapy treatment, and yet the feats kept on coming. In addition to the three London Marathons, they included a full Ironman (2.4-mile swim, 112-mile bike ride and full marathon, completed inside 16 hours), two half-Ironmans, the New York Marathon, three London triathlons and three long-distance bike rides (John O'Groats to Land's End, Rome to Home and her final challenge, a 4,200-mile ride across America).

Tomlinson's illness forced her to retire from competition at the end of 2006, but she devoted her remaining energies to an event which has proved an important part of her legacy, the Leeds 10k Run for All. The first one was held in June 2007 and was a huge success attracting 8,000 participants. Jane sadly lost her battle with cancer just three months later. She died in September 2007, at the age of 43, at which point her efforts had raised more than £1,850,000 for charities including Macmillan Cancer Support, SPARKS, Damon Runyon Cancer Research, Yorkshire Cancer Centre, Martin House Hospice, Bluebell Wood Children's Hospice and Hannah House.

In February 2015, Tomlinson's family confirmed her charity had now raised £7.6 million. Since the first Leeds 10k Run for All in 2007, other fundraising races have followed in York, Sheffield and Hull. Tomlinson's husband, Mike, spoke movingly of the inspiration she offered:

> *If someone has had a cancer diagnosis, they don't have to run a marathon but hopefully her story will give people some hope that diagnosis is not the end of your life. You can still have a fulfilling life.*

Tomlinson received numerous awards along the way including an MBE and subsequently a CBE; the Helen Rollason Award at the BBC Sports Personality of the Year Awards in 2002; and a Great Briton award. In recognition of her work, the laboratory at Cancer Research UK's Clinical Centre at St James's Hospital in Leeds was renamed the Jane Tomlinson Laboratory in 2003, the year she was voted the Most Inspirational Woman in Britain. Two years later she received a Pride of Britain award.

There was further recognition in March 2015 when a plaque was erected in the Victoria Gardens in Leeds, a place which had been a focal point during many of her challenges. The gardens are also the finishing line for the Leeds 10k she founded. Tomlinson proved beyond doubt that there is life to be had after a cancer diagnosis. Her example and achievements continue to inspire people today. Her legacy lives on.

Jane's epic events

End to End Challenge, March 2003	Jane and her brother, Luke Goward, tandem-cycled from Land's End to John O'Groats.
Rome to Home Bike Ride, May 2004	Jane and Luke completed a 36-day tandem ride across Italy, France and England. They raised more than £232,000 in their six-week challenge.

Ironman Florida, November 2004	Jane became the first cancer patient to complete a full Ironman triathlon (2.4-mile swim, 112-mile cycle, 26.2-mile full marathon). She crossed the finish line in a time of 15 hours 47 minutes.
Ride Across America, June 2006	Jane began her biggest fundraising event, a 4,200-mile ride across America, from San Francisco to New York over ten weeks, often over tough terrain including climbs of up to 13,000 feet and desert temperatures of up to 43°C (110°F).

Hyvon Ngetich – A remarkable finish

'You ran the bravest race and crawled the bravest crawl I have ever seen in my life.'
AUSTIN MARATHON RACE DIRECTOR JOHN CONLEY

If you want to know what marathon runners are made of, go to YouTube and search for Hyvon Ngetich. Watch the 29-year-old Kenyan runner cross the finishing line in the 2015 Austin Marathon, and you will almost certainly do so with tears in your eyes. She does so on her hands and knees.

Having led most of the way, Ngetich had her sights set on victory before slipping back into second place. But then with the finish in view, she started to stagger disastrously before collapsing. Ngetich tried and failed to get back up, but even though she couldn't stand, she remained determined to achieve some kind of forward momentum. Several times you can see her pause for breath as she inches agonisingly closer to the finishing line. Medical staff offered her a wheelchair, but Ngetich declined, knowing she would be disqualified if she allowed them to intervene. Having completed the first 26 miles on two legs, she was left with no option but to complete the final two-tenths of a mile on all fours.

With just 2 metres to go, second-place finisher Hannah Steffan passed to push Ngetich back into third place. Across her face, you can see the grim resolution; sadly, you can also see the disorientation. And yet still she made it. 'Oh, God, thank you, I crossed,' she said as she eventually reached the line in 3:04:02.

Race director John Conley, speaking to FOX 7 TV, summed up the thoughts of many:

> *When she came around the corner on her hands and knees, I have never, in 43 years of being involved in this sport, seen a finish like that.*

Ngetich admitted she had absolutely no recollection of the final 2 miles. She was later found to have dangerously low levels of blood sugar.

> *I can't remember what happened, and I didn't see the finish line. I don't remember all that crawling or whatever ... even the collapsing I don't remember.*

But there was no doubting this was Ngetich's day – a day when third place was as good as first, if not better. No one's now watching Cynthia Jerop, the women's winner, cross the line as they settle down to YouTube. Ngetich summed it up when she spoke with KEYE-TV: 'Running, always you have got to keep going, going. You need to die running, you know.'

Eddie Izzard – The comedian who ran his way into the nation's hearts

'This wasn't supposed to be on my list of things to do.'

Eddie Izzard made his name as a transvestite comedian with a strong line in surrealist humour. With a tendency to put on weight, he'd never before run more than 5 miles. But after five weeks of training, he embarked on a journey that was to make him one of the country's least-likely and yet best-loved sporting heroes, completing the equivalent of 43 marathons in just 52 days across the UK – before the comedy once again took over.

Izzard set out on his odyssey on 26 July 2009, taking just one rest day a week and losing a couple of days to travel to Northern Ireland. Otherwise, he ran at least a marathon every day, sometimes as many as 31 miles. Accompanying him was a small support team comprising his tour manager, a sports therapist and an ice-cream van dispensing free ice creams along the way.

Izzard's trek took him from London to Cardiff, Belfast and Edinburgh and eventually deposited him at a point beyond exhaustion. As he told the *Guardian*:

> *If you imagine you drive in a tiny Mini across a wasteland where there is no petrol station and the petrol gauge is always on empty, that is me. I put a little in every night and the needle moves and then the next day I'm below empty again. I am falling asleep when I'm talking to people.*

After more than 1,110 miles, Izzard deserved his glorious finish. On 15 September he dragged his aching body into Trafalgar Square and up the steps in front of the National Gallery. Looking understandably exhausted, he still managed to convey the sheer exhilaration of the moment at the end of a journey that had cemented his place in the nation's hearts. Izzard had hoped to complete his final marathon in less than 5 hours, but he missed his target by 30 seconds – not that anyone seemed to mind. Even by the time he finished, the 47-year-old had already raised more than £200,000 for the Sport Relief charity.

Standing at the finish, he said:

> *Being here is very nice. When I left here seven and a half weeks ago there was nobody here. It was just a cold morning. The worst part of the whole experience was the last 3 minutes sprinting down The Mall. That was really tough.*

He declared his mind was OK, just a bit fuddled and that his priority now was to sleep for a week. Otherwise he was in remarkably good shape. In fact, for many, the most fascinating thing was that Izzard got better as he went on – what sports scientists call, somewhat stating the obvious, 'the training effect'. When he set out, he was completing the daily distance in around 10 hours. By the time he finished, Izzard had halved his time to a little over five. His body adjusted to the physical demands he was putting on it: his muscles enlarged, his heart rate lowered and his lung capacity and breathing improved. 'It's changed my body,' Izzard said.

In March 2016, Izzard once again hit the running headlines when he completed 27 marathons in 27 days in South Africa for Sport Relief – a marathon for every year Nelson Mandela spent in prison before becoming South Africa's first black president.

After being forced to take an unscheduled rest day on the fifth day, 54-year-old Izzard needed to run a double marathon on the final day to complete his challenge beneath a statue of Mandela in Pretoria, the administrative capital of South Africa.

Four years earlier, Izzard was forced to pull out of a similar feat for health reasons. This time, despite dehydration, heat exhaustion and sunstroke, he completed 707 miles to raise more than £1.35 million for Sport Relief. He swigged from a celebratory bottle of sparkling white wine to mark his achievement.

> *That was very, very tough. It's been the hardest thing I've ever done. Thank you to everyone who has donated. Don't do this at home!*

Terry Fox – The Marathon of Hope

'It took cancer to realise that being self-centred is not the way to live. The answer is to try and help others.'

On 30 June 1999 a national survey voted Terry Fox Canada's Greatest Hero, a remarkable accolade for a remarkable man who inspired a nation in his final weeks of life. Even now, his legacy continues to grow. The Terry Fox Run is a non-competitive event where people get together as individuals, families, and groups to raise money for cancer research in Terry's name.

> *I'm not a dreamer, and I'm not saying this will initiate any kind of definitive answer or cure to cancer, but I believe in miracles. I have to.*

Terry Fox (1958–1981) was born in Winnipeg, Manitoba and raised in British Columbia. A sporty teenager, he was just 18 years old when he was diagnosed with bone cancer and had to have his right leg amputated 6 inches above the knee. But it wasn't himself that Fox thought about during his hospital stay. He was overwhelmed by the suffering of his fellow cancer patients, particularly the children. And he decided to do something about it: to become the first person to run across Canada with an artificial leg, as a fundraiser for cancer research. Fox declared it would be his Marathon of Hope.

> *As I went through the 16 months of the physically and emotionally draining ordeal of chemotherapy, I was rudely awakened by the feelings that surrounded and coursed through the cancer clinic. There were faces with the brave smiles, and the ones who had given up smiling. There were feelings of hopeful denial and the feelings*

of despair. My quest would not be a selfish one. I could not leave knowing these faces and feelings would still exist, even though I would be set free from mine. Somewhere the hurting must stop... and I was determined to take myself to the limit for this cause.

Fox's preparation over the next 18 months involved running 5,000 km (3,107 miles) until he felt ready to embark on his big adventure, starting in St John's, Newfoundland on 12 April 1980 – not that many people noticed. It was all decidedly low key. But then the word began to spread. Every day, he would run more or less a marathon distance as he progressed through Canada's provinces, Quebec and Ontario, and as Fox's distance increased, so did interest in his monumental undertaking. And so did the money he was raising.

However, Fox's cancer was starting to spread to his lungs. On 1 September, after 143 days and 5,373 km (3,339 miles), breathless and in pain, he was forced to stop running. By now he was big news, and the $1.7 million he had raised at that point soon grew. Fundraisers multiplied as Fox underwent chemotherapy – all to no avail. He died on 28 June 1981, at the age of 22.

In many ways, Fox's death was simply the beginning. A nation responded. Canada embraced his courage and took his spirit to its heart. So far, more than $650 million has been raised worldwide for cancer research in his name.

I don't feel that this is unfair. That's the thing about cancer. I'm not the only one, it happens all the time to people. I'm not special. This just intensifies what I did. It gives it more meaning. It'll inspire more people. I just wish people would realise that anything's possible if you try. Dreams are made possible if you try.

Terry Fox Runs happen in more than 9,000 communities across Canada every year. The whole point is that they are accessible to everyone. There is no entry fee and there is no minimum pledge, and participants can run, walk, rollerblade or bike. The only thing that matters is that they have fun while raising funds for cancer research. Every single Terry Fox Run celebrates Terry's legacy; each run helps to keep alive his hope that a cure for cancer will be found.

Recognition for Terry Fox in the years following his death

17 July 1981	British Columbia names a 2,639-m peak in the Rocky Mountains Mount Terry Fox.
30 July 1981	An 83-km section of the Trans-Canada Highway is renamed the Terry Fox Courage Highway.
30 July 1981	The Canadian government creates a $5 million endowment fund named the Terry Fox Humanitarian Award to provide scholarships each year.

29 August 1981	Fox is posthumously inducted into the Canadian Sports Hall of Fame.
13 September 1981	The first Terry Fox Run is held at more than 760 sites in Canada and around the world, attracting 300,000 participants and raising $3.5 million.
13 April 1982	Canada Post issues a Terry Fox Stamp.
December 1990	The Sports Network names Terry Fox Athlete of the Decade.
11 February 1994	The Terry Fox Hall of Fame is created to recognise Canadians who have made extraordinary personal contributions to the lives of people with physical disabilities.

Bruce Cleland – The world's first charity runner

'It's a programme for people with really big hearts.'

For millions of marathoners around the world, a key part of their motivation as they churn out the 26.2 miles is the thought of the charity they are running for. For many, it is a huge part of the reason they are doing it in the first place. But it wasn't always this way. It took a special person in a moment of personal crisis to see the massive fundraising potential every single marathon can unlock. That man was Bruce Cleland, a marathoner regarded by many as the world's first charity runner.

It all began in 1986 when Cleland's two-year-old daughter, Georgia, was diagnosed with leukaemia. He was convinced it was the end.

> *In a word, it was terrifying. At that time, whenever I heard someone had leukaemia, it was usually a death sentence. In those days the survival rate was only about 5 per cent.*

However, Cleland and his wife, Izzi, soon learnt that the long-term survival rate for childhood leukaemia was a much more promising 55 per cent. The world of childhood blood cancer became their world as they tried to make sense of all the treatments their daughter now faced. Crucial support came from the Leukemia Society of America, now known as the Leukemia & Lymphoma Society or LLS. Two years later, Georgia was in remission.

The family had been doing all the usual fundraising activities, but it was at this point that Cleland had an idea. A marathon. Something different. Something usually considered beyond mere mortals. Something special. The idea soon gathered pace, and Team in Training was born (www.teamintraining.org), a flagship fundraising programme for LLS and the only endurance sports initiative which raises money for blood cancer research.

For the 1988 New York City Marathon, Cleland put a team together. Thirty-eight runners raised $322,000 for LLS's work to discover new treatments for blood cancers. A new tradition of giving had taken root – one very much at the heart of thousands of big marathons now.

In the nearly 30 years since, LLS's Team in Training (TNT) has funded significant therapies, which have included chemotherapy and bone marrow transplants. The result has been a direct and significant impact on blood cancer patients. The figures are remarkable. Since 1988, more than 600,000 TNT participants have helped LLS invest more than $1 billion into blood cancer research. For Cleland, the joy is that Georgia herself has become one of those participants. For years cancer-free, she completed her first half-marathon in 2012 to raise funds for Team in Training.

For Cleland, it's about being part of a team working towards a greater goal:

> *I was one of these middle-age people who could remember the thrill of being part of a team. I don't think you ever forget. It's such a special part of your life. You knock the stuffing out of the guy or whatever it is you're supposed to do. Those are the stories you remember and the people you remember. You move past it, but you remember that feeling.*

Guiding it all, though, is the difference Team in Training is making. Today, the survival rate for two-year-olds diagnosed with acute lymphoblastic leukaemia is above 90 per cent.

Ironically, Cleland is himself now a survivor. He was diagnosed with stage IV throat cancer. Radiation and chemotherapy failed to eradicate it, and eventually his life was saved by a 17-and-a-half-hour operation. Two years later and cancer-free, he celebrated by completing the 2008 Baltimore Marathon in 6 hours 3 minutes.

Jennifer Sheridan – 'Be good, be strong'

'I realised there was something I could do to help'

Every year the Massachusetts General Hospital Cancer Center honours 100 'Everyday Amazing' individuals and groups — caregivers, researchers, philanthropists, advocates and volunteers from around the globe — whose commitment to the fight against cancer inspires everyone else not just to take notice, but to take action. As the centre explains, the idea is to offer hope, inspire action and show how we can fight cancer together.

Among the nominees in 2012 was committed runner Jennifer Sheridan who had lost two sisters and a brother to cancer. During their illness, Sheridan and the rest of the family shared responsibility for their care. She took them to doctors' appointments and even moved her brother in during his chemotherapy – all while raising three young children with her husband.

> *I am inspired by my siblings Milly, Mary and John, all of whom lost their lives to cancer as young adults. I am inspired by the way they lived their lives with hope and strength and always fighting the good fight.*

A turning point came when Sheridan watched the 2008 Boston Marathon. She realised it was potentially an outlet for her grief and also a way she might channel her desire to help. Just a couple of months earlier, in February 2008, her sister Molly Firth-Hooper had died of cancer at the age of 36. Her brother John and sister Mary were also struggling against the disease.

> *Back on the April day in 2008, as I watched all of those runners pass by, still feeling so much grief from Molly's death, carrying so much stress and sadness for the ongoing health battle that John and Mary continued to face, I realised there was something I could do to help. I could run while raising money for cancer research.*

Sheridan ran her first Boston Marathon in 2009 in memory of Molly. She also ran it in honour of her brother John who had an almost identical brain tumour to the one that had killed their sister. With their names printed on her shirt, Sheridan paused on the course to hug and kiss friends and family before seeking out John, by then too weak to stand. He died 26 days after the race at the age of 32. In 2010, Sheridan was running the Boston Marathon in his memory too. Their sister Mary died of melanoma a year later, at the age of 35 – three deaths in three years.

In their plight, Sheridan found her own strength. In four years, she raised more than $100,000 for cancer research.

Sheridan runs for the Dana-Farber Marathon Challenge team. The team aims to raise critical funds to benefit the Claudia Adams Barr Program in Innovative Basic Cancer Research at the Dana-Farber Cancer Institute, a world-renowned cancer treatment and research centre in Boston. Since taking its first steps in 1990, DFMC has raised more than $74 million, resulting in improved survival rates and quality of life for cancer patients everywhere. The largest charity group in the Boston Marathon, the 2016 DFMC team aims to raise $5.4 million in pursuit of what it calls the ultimate finish line: a world without cancer.

Looking back, Sheridan didn't know how else to cope. The only way to clear her head was to run, she recalls:

> *Distance-wise it was a gradual thing, commitment-wise, the amount I did it, I was like 'I'm just going to run.' But after doing it the first time I felt better. It was a stress release, a really therapeutic time; time on my own to process things, not talk to anybody.*

'Be good, be strong' was the maxim the family adopted during its darkest hours. It is also the name of Sheridan's blog, the channel through which she offers 'thoughts and opinions on family, running, friends, the sunshine and the snow, cancer, cures, and trying to make a difference. And whatever else comes to mind.'

CHAPTER THREE

THE PIONEERS OF WOMEN'S DISTANCE RUNNING

Violet Piercy – A true pioneer of women's running

*'I did it to prove that a woman's stamina
can be just as remarkable as a man's.'*

An Englishwoman, Paula Radcliffe, currently holds the world
record for the fastest women's marathon, 2:15:25 set in London
in 2003. She was following in the footsteps of Violet Piercy, the
first Englishwoman to attempt a marathon and the first to be
officially timed when she ran 3:40:22 on 3 October 1926 on the
Polytechnic Marathon course between Windsor and London – a
time which stood as an unofficial world record for the next 37 years

until American Merry Lepper ran a time of 3:37:07 in California's Western Hemisphere Marathon on 16 December 1963.

And yet, Piercy fell into obscurity. Peter Lovesey, an athletics historian and award-winning crime novelist, has been instrumental in finally securing for her the recognition she deserves:

> *Stories had been around for a long time about a Londoner called Violet Piercy who ran the marathon in the 1920s when the rules barred any woman from running more than two laps. The* Dictionary of National Biography *asked me to investigate, and I soon found online some Pathé newsreel of her running in 1927. This encouraged me to discover more. Not only did Violet run the marathon five times between 1926 and 1936, but she did it each time in a pair of walking shoes with cross-straps and heels.*

The Pathé newsreel is delightful to watch, giving a priceless insight into a runner who really was from a different era. Piercy can be seen running in a white jersey and black shorts, her running shoes looking more like ballet shoes than anything we might use today. She is accompanied by three cyclists and followed by a car before the location switches to an athletics track. The camera closes in on her feet as she skips as part of her training. Piercy then runs around an athletics track, and we see her run past the camera in slow motion. Finally, she smiles at the camera.

Clearly she had no fear of the limelight. Lively discussion about her achievements among NUTS – the National Union of Track Statisticians – includes a comment from Andy Milroy: 'If she were alive and flourishing today she would be an ideal candidate for *I'm A Celebrity – Get Me Out Of Here!'*

Bizarre, then, that her identity has never been definitively established, maybe because in later life she fell on hard times and no one seems to have any clear information as to what happened to her. The debate continues with five possible contenders in the frame. However, as Peter Lovesey says, all the available evidence indicates a strong probability that she was Violet Stewart Louisa Piercy, who was born in Croydon, Surrey, on 24 December 1889. If this particular Violet Piercy really is the marathon runner, as Lovesey observes, then her achievements were all the more remarkable considering she was 36 at the time of her first distance run and 46 when she indisputably ran 26 miles 385 yards.

> *I am about the only long-distance woman runner in this country, and people rather shout at me about it. I really don't see why they should. Running is about the healthiest form of exercise a woman can have, especially in these days of the slimming craze.*

Through his researches, Lovesey has been able to capture something of her character:

> *She was a doctor's secretary, a buoyant character who blithely broke the rules of the WAAA [Women's Amateur Athletics Association] and broadcast an account of it on the BBC. She did her best to encourage others to do the same, but*

no one took up the challenge in her lifetime, so her runs were solo, except one when she was allowed to start before the men in the annual Windsor to White City race. Even the women athletes in her club thought of her as an oddball. The truth is that she was a generation ahead of everyone else.

Dale Greig – Followed by an ambulance

'I never considered myself as championing women's rights. I ran because I loved being outdoors.'

Think of the undulations along the way on the Isle of Wight Marathon, and it seems one of the least likely places for a world record to be set. But then again, everything was strange about the race which Scottish runner Dale Greig (*b.* 1937) completed on 23 May 1964 – a race which made her the first woman to run a marathon in under 3 hours 30 minutes.

Women were not allowed to run marathons at the time. The thinking was that nice women did not run – thinking enshrined in the early history of the modern Olympics. Women were banned. Baron Pierre de Coubertin, founder of the modern Olympic Games in 1896, made his feelings quite clear:

> *It is indecent that the spectators should be exposed to the risk of seeing the body of a woman being smashed before their very eyes. Besides, no matter how*

> *toughened a sportswoman may be, her organism*
> *is not cut out to sustain certain shocks.*

Women's track and field events were introduced into the 1928 Olympics, but only up to 800 m. Several women collapsed, and the limit was consequently reduced to 100 m, a ceiling that wasn't lifted until the women's 200-m race was introduced in 1948. The 1964 games saw women compete in 100-, 200-, 400- and 800-m races, but still the marathon was unthinkable, at least as far as the Olympic Games were concerned.

And so it was for British athletics as well. In the 1964 Isle of Wight Marathon, Greig had to strike a compromise simply to start. She was made to set off 4 minutes ahead of the men so that she wasn't officially part of the field. So low were the expectations that she would finish, an ambulance followed her round. Afterwards, the Women's Amateur Athletic Association reprimanded the organisers for allowing her to take part in the first place.

Greig, who lives in Paisley, was most definitely a pioneer in women's running, but her efforts received little fanfare. Not that she minded, as she told the *Independent* in an interview in 1997:

> *Life is all about timing, about being in the right place at the right time. I just ran for fun and I don't regret that at all. I really enjoyed it. It just happens to be a different sport now. There was never any thought of making money in those days and, running in the marathon or the London-to-Brighton, it was just a matter of getting round the course. Today the women are racing these distances, racing really fast. I must say I admire them.*

There was no official record Greig could claim at the time, simply a 'best' in an unrecognised event. Her time of 3:27:45 was acknowledged as the fastest recorded by a woman for the standard marathon distance of 26 miles 385 yards. It was bettered a month later when the New Zealander Mildred Sampson clocked 3:19:33 in the Auckland Marathon, but Greig's 'best' stood as a British 'record' for 11 years. Her time is now recognised retrospectively as probably the first reliable world record for women at this distance.

Greig was Scottish Universities' 440-yards champion in 1956 and won four Scottish cross-country titles. She was also the first woman to complete the Ben Nevis race and the Isle of Man 40-mile race over the TT circuit. She broke new ground again in 1972 as the first woman to complete the 55-mile London-to-Brighton race, finishing in 8 hours 30 minutes – seven years before female competitors were officially allowed to enter. Just as in Ryde eight years before, she had to start on her own, an hour before the other runners – simply because women were not allowed to run with men. Greig set off with a map in her hand so she didn't get lost. Two years later, she won the inaugural women's marathon at the world veterans' championships in Paris.

Such talents these days would certainly make her a wealthy woman in athletics. Not so back then. But again, Greig is far from bitter about it all:

> *I am not envious. We ran just for the fun of it. I never made a penny, and I was proud to be an amateur. That's not to say I would not have liked to make a living as a runner, but I believed in the amateur code and actually gave away my prizes. Now it's professional and completely different.*

Dale Greig's achievements

Scottish Universities' 440-yards champion	1956
Scottish cross-country champion	1960, 1962, 1964, 1968
Scottish cross-country internationalist	1957–1970
World record holder women's marathon	1964
First woman to run the Isle of Man TT mountain course (40 miles)	1971
Ran up and down Ben Nevis (4,400 feet)	1971
First woman to run the London-to-Brighton race (55 miles)	1972
IGAL World Champion women's marathon, Paris	1974

Bobbi Gibb – Joining the men

'I did it in order to prove that women could run 26.2 miles and to call into question every other false belief about women.'

Wearing an oversized sweater to conceal her gender and hiding in a clump of bushes near the starting pen, Roberta 'Bobbi' Gibb readied herself for one of the most significant runs ever run by a woman. When the gun went off, she let about half the pack go by before jumping in amongst the hundreds of men streaming past. Her actions were in clear defiance of the Boston Athletic Association. Twenty-six point two miles and 3 hours 21 minutes later, she was the first woman ever to run their marathon.

> *As soon as you became an adolescent, everything changed. You started to become a woman and suddenly there were all these incredible constraints. I could see coming down the line that I was going to have to live in a box as a woman – literally, locked up in the house. We were expected to be housewives, and that's all... We weren't expected to have minds, and we weren't expected to have bodies that ran.*

The day was 19 April 1966, an era when the received wisdom was that women simply weren't capable of running marathons: they would expire long before the end. Gibb (*b.* 1942) didn't see it that way. For her, running was quite simply a natural instinct, a spiritual thing – a chance to get away from society and its rigid thinking. It was a freedom.

However, growing up in the 1950s, she soon realised that it was one of the many freedoms that were going to be curtailed once she moved into adulthood. Gibb began to see it all as part of the unthinking, unreasonable limitations imposed on women generally. At the University of California, San Diego, she enrolled for pre-med until: 'They told me I was too pretty and I'd upset the boys in the lab.' Things had to change, and Gibb was going to play her part.

> *That's what everyone thought. I mean, this was a universal truth. Women can't be doctors, it's too much stress. Women can't be lawyers, it's too much stress. Women can't be in the government... women can't run long distance. Women can't do anything except stay home and clean the house. It was like being in a cage. It was horrible... It was just everywhere. It was ubiquitous.*

Gibb, who was born and raised in Massachusetts, watched the Boston Marathon for the first time in 1964. She believed she had found running's greatest expression and determined to run it. It was only later that she realised that she would be making a social statement. Prevailing thinking told her that 26.2 miles might kill her, but with no one to guide her and no idea how to train, she tested the distance bit by bit as she prepared for the big day, never knowing quite what was going to happen, but always pushing her abilities as the marathon approached. She managed 40 miles in one practice run.

Gibb was ready but her application to run the Boston Marathon was rejected – for the simple reason that she was a woman and therefore could not possibly compete safely. She was enraged and resolved to run it anyway. It was no longer just a run: it was a question of combating ignorant, prejudiced thinking. As she later said, someone had to 'blow the whole thing wide open'; she resolved to 'throw into question all the other prejudices and misconceptions that were used to keep women down for centuries'. The marathon was suddenly so much more than a running race.

And so she sneaked in among the runners, wearing her brother's Bermuda shorts, a pair of boys' trainers, a bathing suit and a sweatshirt. She feared arrest, but once it became clear that other runners actually welcomed a woman in their midst and would protect her, she felt safe to take off her sweatshirt.

> *We got talking and they said: 'Gee, I wish my girlfriend would run. I wish my wife would run.' They wanted to share their love of running with the women in their lives.*

The crowd was instantly behind her in a huge emotional outburst. Men were cheering and clapping; women were jumping up and down wildly and weeping. Word spread. And in Gibb's mind the responsibility grew. She knew she had to finish. She realised the damage failure to finish would do to the cause she was now running for.

> *I was actually running way slower than I wanted to. I was saving my energy because I knew that the worst thing that could happen would be if I didn't finish. I had this huge weight of responsibility on me. Here I was, making this very public statement. If I had collapsed or hadn't finished, I would have set women back another 50 years or maybe longer.*

Gibb came home one hundred and twenty-sixth overall, a top-third finish, and the governor of Massachusetts John Volpe was there at the end to shake her hand. No longer the only woman, she ran the race again in 1967 and 1968. Gibb claimed the unofficial women's title both years.

In 1968, five women ran in all, all without the official numbers that were denied them. Pressure for change was beginning to grow. Gibb's view was that she was opening people's minds. It was an important contribution to the women's movement of the 1960s.

> *I see women running and they look so strong and confident. I feel like they're all my daughters. That's the reason I did all this – so women could feel strong and confident.*

Kathrine Switzer – A pioneer of women's marathon running

'I looked square into the most vicious face I'd ever seen.'

Few women have been more influential in women's running than Kathrine Switzer, an athlete who really did change the face of the sport.

Bobbi Gibb set the ball rolling for women's marathon running in 1966; Switzer took things to the next level on the same Boston course in 1967. Gibb was the first woman to run the Boston Marathon; Switzer was the first woman to register to run it – and the resulting photographs still shock today. Switzer was physically attacked by the race director for wearing an official race number – a moment captured in images which flashed around the globe to become one of *Time-Life*'s 100 Photos that Changed the World.

Switzer used to sign her college papers K V Switzer and did so when she registered for the all-male Boston Marathon in 1967. She wasn't the first woman to run the race, but the fact that she was apparently there as an official entrant was a red rag to the race authorities when they saw her on the course. Boston Athletic Association official Jock Semple wasn't having it. In her book, *Marathon Woman*, Switzer recalls:

> *I heard the scraping noise of leather shoes coming up fast behind me, an alien and alarming sound amid the muted thump thumping of rubber-soled running shoes. When a runner hears that kind of noise, it's usually danger — like hearing a dog's paws on the pavement. Instinctively I jerked my head around quickly and looked square into the most vicious face I'd ever seen. A big man, a huge man, with bared teeth was set to pounce, and before I could react he grabbed my shoulder and flung me back, screaming, 'Get the hell out of my race and give me those numbers!' Then he swiped down my front, trying to rip off my bib number, just as I leapt backward from him.*

Switzer's boyfriend, an ex-All-American football player, intervened and took Semple out with a body block. It was just 4 miles in; Switzer's coach told her to 'Run like hell!' Looking back, Switzer sees it as the transformative moment in her life, the moment she was radicalised. Fear was replaced with resolve.

> " *I just doubled down and became very, very, very determined to finish the race no matter what because I knew suddenly it wasn't just about running. It was about proving that women deserved to be there and could be there.*

Switzer carried that weight for the next 22 miles. She crossed the line an hour after Bobbi Gibb, but it was Switzer who stole the headlines. Her finish fanned the fire Gibb had started. Five years later, women were officially allowed to enter the Boston Marathon. In 1972, eight women started and finished.

Two years later, in 1974, Switzer was the women's winner in the New York City Marathon. She then clocked a personal best in 1975, finishing second (2:51:33) on the same Boston course she'd been attacked on. She went on to run 39 marathons in all before focusing her energies on creating the Avon International Running Circuit of women-only races in 27 countries.

Switzer has continued to show that running is all about bringing people together. In effect, as she says, the worst experience in her life became the best experience for all that it brought with it. She later became 'best of friends' with Jock Semple; but more importantly, she has watched what running has done for women. For Switzer and her successors, it has been about empowerment, about changing lives for the better. It has also been about changing perceptions as we move towards a greater understanding of women's capabilities. For women, Switzer triggered a greater belief in those capabilities – to the extent that it is estimated that 58 per cent of all runners in the United States are now women.

Switzer's place in running history has been to show that you can change everything – simply by putting one foot in front of the other.

Named Runner of the Decade (1966–76), Switzer was also named one of the Visionaries of the Century (2000) and a Hero of Running (2012) by *Runner's World* magazine. She stands as a force for social change in running. Switzer was instrumental in getting the International Olympic Committee to include a women's marathon in the 1984 Olympic Games, but her influence goes far beyond the elite runners. Millions of women around the world have been encouraged to run by Switzer's example, to the point where the activity has become a social revolution. Seeing this, Switzer has recently created '261 Fearless'. Named after the old bib number that the race official tried to tear off her, '261 Fearless' is a non-profit organisation that aims to bring together, encourage and empower female runners.

Thirty-eight years after those infamous photographs flashed around the world, 13,374 women stood on the start line in the 2015 Boston Marathon. Every single one was, of course, an official entrant. Switzer had won.

Miki Gorman – Conquering the doubts

'I left Japan with $10 in my pocket. I still have the passport. And now I can live comfortably. I'm proud of that.'

The general feeling is that Miki Gorman was ahead of her time. If that's the case, then it's safe to say that time still hasn't caught up with her, 40 years after her greatest running feats.

Hailed as the 'Runner of the 1970s' by the New York Road Runners in 2009, Gorman remains the only woman to have won both the New York City and Boston marathons twice. She is also one of only two women to win Boston and New York in the same year.

Gorman's achievements are seen as important stepping stones along the way towards the present-day complete acceptance of women's long-distance running. But it must be remembered that she was running in an era where the doubts persisted still.

Born Michiko Suwa in 1935 to Japanese parents in occupied China, she endured hardship and hunger in her early years. After World War Two, the family settled north of Tokyo where times were tough.

Miki moved to the United States in 1964 at the age of 28 to take secretarial classes at Carlisle Commercial College in Pennsylvania. She later moved to Los Angeles and married. Gorman took up running in 1968 and at first was a reluctant runner. Soon she became a triumphant one, always ignoring any niggling and offensive suggestions that she really ought to be back home in the kitchen.

Gorman recalled:

> My husband pushed me into running because my social life was very limited. I tried exercise class, but it was boring. I enjoyed running, although I sometimes got dirty looks because I was a woman running.

A late starter, Gorman, just 5 feet tall, set an unofficial world best marathon time of 2:46:36 in 1973 at the Western Hemisphere Marathon, now the Culver City Marathon. Much better was yet to come. She won the Boston Marathon in 1974 and won it again in 1977. In between times, she triumphed in the New York City Marathon in consecutive years, winning in 1976 and

1977, at the age of 41 and 42. These were golden years for the diminutive champion who remained modest to the end. When she was inducted into the National Distance Running Hall of Fame in 2010, she said simply: 'I do not deserve it.' Injuries forced her to give up marathons in 1978.

Gorman died in September 2015, in Bellingham, Washington, at the age of 80 after battling cancer for five years. The Boston Athletic Association, organisers of the Boston Marathon, were among the many to pay tribute:

> *Miki inspired women of all ages and backgrounds to run. She was a leader during the early years of women's marathoning.*

'I don't know if I'm proud. A friend tells me I should be, but I'm not really. Those times were pretty slow, compared to today. My dream was to become a violinist. But my father never spent any money on me because I was a girl. So I didn't become a musician. If I'm proud of my running, it's that I did my best and I worked hard. I was in my 40s. If I was younger, I'm sure I could have run faster.' *New York Times*

Miki Gorman's marathon successes

1973	Culver City Marathon	1st place, 2:46:36 (WR)
1974	Boston Marathon	1st place, 2:47:11
1975	New York City Marathon	2nd place, 2:53:02
1976	Boston Marathon	2nd place, 2:52:27
1976	New York City Marathon	1st place, 2:39:11
1977	Boston Marathon	1st place, 2:48:33
1977	New York City Marathon	1st place, 2:43:11

CHAPTER FOUR
BECAUSE IT'S THERE

Dave McGillivray – The race director who runs his years

*'To be involved in arguably the greatest marathon
in the world is a unique and coveted privilege.'*

On the morning of his twelfth birthday, Dave McGillivray took off on a run from his home in Massachusetts, a 6-mile loop which he repeated later that day, 22 August 1966. The following year he ran 13 miles on his thirteenth birthday; the year after that, 14 on his fourteenth birthday. And so it has continued. Unbroken.

McGillivray freely confesses he has allowed his own rules to evolve. The runs don't have to be continuous, and for his fortieth birthday, he ran his 40 miles the day before so as not to interfere with a big party.

As the years started to mount up, McGillivray admits he has started to agonise about his ever-growing challenge. After he turned 50, he thought about going in reverse. For every birthday starting at

51, he thought he'd take a mile off. At 51, he'd do 49, then 48 at 52 and so on. The reasoning was that for his seventieth, he'd have to do only 30 miles. But McGillivray didn't like the reasoning when it came to putting it into practice. On his fifty-first birthday run, he stopped at 49 miles, just as he intended. But he didn't know what to do next. He resolved the dilemma by running another 2 miles. Fifty-one for his fifty-first, and he was back on track.

'My game, my rules. That's my motto,' he said as he approached the big one, his sixtieth. But he managed it. Starting 3.5-mile loops from his house from 2 a.m., he calculated he would finish at about 4.30 p.m., an hour and a half before his birthday party. In fact, he finished at 4.15 p.m. – even better for the celebration ahead.

And so the years keep on coming. McGillivray confesses an option one day might be to convert miles to kilometres. But he's not there yet.

However, it's not for his birthday runs that McGillivray is best known. Nor is it for the fact that in 1978, he ran from Medford, Oregon to Medford, Massachusetts, a total of 3,452 miles, to raise thousands of dollars for the Jimmy Fund and the Dana-Farber Cancer Institute. Nor even is it for the fact that in 1982, he ran a 3-hour 14-minute marathon blindfolded to raise more than $10,000 for the Carroll Center for the Blind.

For millions, it is the Boston Marathon that is Dave McGillivray's greatest claim to fame. He has been the race director since 1988 and has another set of traditions he likes to maintain as part of his involvement, namely taking part – after the event.

In 2013, the year of the Boston bombing, McGillivray ran the course 11 days after the race had completed. McGillivray, who boasts a 2:29:58 marathon personal best and has completed more than 130 marathons, had other things on his mind that day – just as he had when the race returned in 2014 for its first year back after the bombing. He conceded it would be a very different marathon. The logistics of putting on one of the world's highest-profile races had been transformed, and McGillivray knew the world would be watching. Despite his understandable anxiety, everything passed off successfully.

In April 2015, McGillivray ran his forty-third consecutive Boston Marathon. Remarkably, he ran 27 of the most recent 28 at night after completing his duties as race director. For McGillivray, 2015 was a particularly tough one. He completed the course in pouring rain with six friends, the last of the 26,610 official finishers in the one hundred and nineteenth running of the race.

Amy Hughes – 53 marathons in 53 days

'I feel like I can keep going. If anything I feel stronger.'

Twenty-six-year-old sports therapist Amy Hughes put theory into practice when she completed 53 marathons in as many days in September 2014, securing her place in the record books. She started in Chester on 6 August and ended in Manchester on 27 September. If someone had suggested a fifty-fourth marathon, she quipped, she would probably have gone for it.

Hughes ran her way through five pairs of trainers as she clocked up 1,389 miles in all, running in cities including London, Liverpool, Wolverhampton, Newcastle, Glasgow and Cardiff. Support was particularly strong when she completed marathon number 50 in her home town of Oswestry in Shropshire. Paula Radcliffe was among the many to get behind her efforts, tweeting her support for Amy's 'amazing and inspirational accomplishment'. Her efforts were also lauded by Manchester United and England footballer Wayne

Rooney, who praised her 'great achievement' on Twitter. As for rewards along the way, Hughes confessed to jelly babies, Percy Pig sweets and chocolate bars.

A low point came on the thirty-fifth day when a stomach bug meant she was sick and suffered painful stomach cramps. But determination and support from friends and onlookers kept her going.

Hughes set out with a double mission, partly to encourage children to be more active, partly also to raise money for the Isabelle Lottie Foundation after a friend's daughter was diagnosed with a brain tumour. Hughes managed to raise more than £40,000. She wrote on her fundraising website, www.53marathons.co.uk:

> *I was and still am overwhelmed by the amount of positive feedback and support I received throughout my challenge and after the event. The messages and donations made have been incredible. To think I have inspired and reached out to so many makes me smile every day.*

Hughes says her life has been a whirlwind since completing her challenge. She has kept busy as a personal trainer, sports therapist and nutrition coach, but she has also worked with a number of companies and campaigns, including an appearance on BBC's *Blue Peter*. She has also started working with the Dame Kelly Holmes Trust, which supports athletes as they transition from sport and also helps them use their skills to transform the lives of disadvantaged young people through mentoring programmes.

Kim Allan – Three and a half days without sleep

'Someone get this Iron Woman a pillow.'
NEW YORK DAILY NEWS

In December 2013, New Zealand ultradistance runner Kim Allan ran her way into the record books with a run that almost defies belief. She broke the world record for running without sleep, covering 500 km (311 miles) in 86 hours, all without a mere hint of a nod, let alone a doze.

The triumph was all the sweeter for the fact she had tried before and failed. The year before, Allan abandoned a record bid after suffering from hallucinations and losing all her toe nails.

> *In all honesty, it's just mental discipline. You've just got to get your head around it. Which is all good and well but unfortunately last year when it got on to the last day, when I had been awake for 80 hours, I had no idea why I was here. I didn't know what I was doing and why these people were making me walk, and I was saying to them, 'This is insane. Who would make an event where you're not allowed to sleep? That's just dumb.' Then I thought I was in France doing some adventure trail event!*

For Allan, it was a double celebration when she finally achieved her goal in 2013. Raising money for the New Zealand Spinal Trust, which supports people with spinal injuries, she passed the previous women's record of 486 km (302 miles) for running without sleep and went on to reach her 500 km (311 miles) goal just over 2 hours later, the point at which she finally stopped. To be precise, she had run for 86 hours 11 minutes 9 seconds.

> *To be honest, going out on a 2-hour training run is just a drag. There's ultrarunners who go out and train huge miles. That's not me. It's the beating my own mind that I like. Thinking you can't do something, then you go out and do it.*

The 47-year-old mother of four, a vegetarian and former jockey, achieved the feat by completing 332 laps of a circuit in Auckland. Allan started her run on a Thursday at about 6 a.m. and finished on the Sunday night. Along the way she had to cut the tops of her shoes off to relieve her blisters. At the end, her team described her as overwhelmed but 'cognitive'.

Achim Aretz – Putting your best foot backwards!

> *'When [I] run backwards*
> *for 20 or 30 kilometres,*
> *sometimes I feel that I fly.'*

Children used to chase him; adults settled for simply asking why, but for Germany's Achim Aretz, running backwards was just as natural as running forwards – so natural in fact that he ran himself backwards into the record books twice. Aretz has completed both the world's fastest backwards half-marathon and the world's fastest backwards full marathon.

Aretz chanced on running backwards – sometimes called retro-running – when he woke up with a hangover. To shake it off, he went for a run with a friend. Because Aretz was so slow, his friend opted to run backwards. Aretz joined in; backwards running took over; and Aretz started competing as a retro-runner. Aretz always insisted it was safer than it looked and that he had fallen only once. The attraction wasn't the possible danger. It was the mental challenge, plus the fact he was developing different muscles to the runners who run forwards.

> When I am running alone, I have to look back maybe every 10 metres, and when I am running together with friends, they can tell me what lies behind me and they can warn me.

Medical specialists have confirmed that running backwards allows better recovery from certain knee, ankle and groin injuries. Running backwards will also apparently burn more calories but with 20 per cent less effort than running forwards. In a blog for the reverse running website, *StrideUK*, performance analyst Mitchell Phillips underlined the benefits he believed walking or running backwards brings, describing it as a great way to cool down, and also to improve balance and increase neuromuscular efficiency. For Phillips, it is the perfect remedy to help 'cure the frequent deficiency between anterior and posterior chain muscle groups – the hamstrings/calves and quads'.

In his book, *Backwards Running*, Robert K. Stevenson goes further, describing it as a fantastic way to train your body and an outstanding activity for physical conditioning.

Stevenson was writing at a time when retro-running was starting to gain popularity, but a number of serious athletes had been using it for years as part of their training regime, among them early twentieth century athletes including boxer Gene Tunney and wrestling champions William Muldoon and Ed Schultz.

However, even Aretz eventually reached the point where he felt he wanted to turn and face the front. Mission accomplished, in 2012 at the age of 27, Aretz announced he was giving up retro-running. He had achieved all he set out to achieve and wanted a new direction – forwards.

Running backwards records

Half-marathon		
7 August 1987	Yves Pol (FRA)	1:42:00
28 November 2009	Achim Aretz (DEU)	1:40:29
28 May 2011	Achim Aretz (DEU)	1:35:49

Marathon		
26 October 1980	Ernest C Conner Jr (USA)	5:18:00
3 October1982	Anthony Weiland (USA)	4:07:54
February 1985	Albert Freese (USA)	3:59:07
16 September 1987	Yves Pol (FRA)	3:57:56
13 May 1990	Yves Pol (FRA)	3:57:26

24 April 1994	Bud Badyna (USA)	3:53:17
17 October 2004	Xu Zhenjun (CHN)	3:43:39
31 October 2010	Achim Aretz (DEU)	3:42:41

Fiona Oakes – The meat-free athlete

'Veganism is everything to me.'

You know you're tough when they think you're tough in Siberia. In fact, they think Fiona Oakes is tough pretty much everywhere. To her credit is a remarkable succession of races, all run to demonstrate the total, natural viability of the vegan lifestyle.

She told the *Viva La Vegan* website in 2012:

> *[Veganism] touches every part of my life. It is my life. I could not begin to imagine living my life any other way. It's not just the diet, but the lifestyle and the life choices I have made through my veganism, such as starting the Tower Hill Stables Animal Sanctuary and my marathon running.*

As a vegan for more than 40 years, she participates in endurance sport to demonstrate that her diet is not prohibitive to performance. The results speak for themselves. In 2012, Oakes became the first life-long vegan female to complete the gruelling Marathon des Sables, a race often styled the toughest footrace on the planet: a marathon a day for six days across the Sahara Desert, carrying all your supplies on your back. Fiona completed the race again in 2014.

With more than 50 marathons under her belt and a personal best of 2 hours 38 minutes, Oakes holds no fewer than five marathon course records – the Essex Championship Marathon, the Dartmoor Vale Marathon, the Ruska Marathon, the Antarctic Ice Marathon and the North Pole Marathon.

Her statistics are astonishing. In 2013, Oakes became the fastest woman in history to run a marathon on all seven continents in terms of the total number of hours taken. She is also the fastest woman to run a marathon on all seven continents plus the North Pole – both in terms of the aggregate time and the elapsed days – and all despite the loss of a kneecap to illness in her early teenage years. In 2014, Oakes was a finalist in the Vegan Athlete of the Year competition.

She told the *Great Vegan Athletes* website:

> I like to encourage people to think about veganism in a positive way.
> I try to break down stereotypes and myths attached to veganism by my actions. I am one of only 800 female fire-fighters in the UK – a job which people don't expect to see a female doing, let alone a vegan one. I run endurance events, a thing which people don't think you can do if you are a 'weak vegan'.

Oakes sees it all as putting into practice her belief that the body can get all it needs from a plant-based lifestyle; she argues it's a realisation that more and more of us will need to make 'if we are to salvage the environment as well as bring to an end the suffering, misery and slaughter faced by billions of animals every year'.

Originally from Chesterfield, Oakes puts her beliefs into practice at the Tower Hill Stables Animal Sanctuary in Essex, which provides a home to around 350 rescued animals – both domestic and ex-farm. She also created the Fiona Oakes Foundation to promote what she sees as the single biggest issue facing the world in which we live: sustainability.

Oakes' world records, all achieved in 2013

Fastest woman to run a marathon on each continent	Aggregate time 23:27:40
Fastest woman to run a marathon on each continent plus the North Pole	Aggregate time 28:20:50
Fastest woman to run a marathon on each continent plus the North Pole	Elapsed time 225 days

Jon Sutherland – The greatest, unbroken running streak

'The first thing I think about when I wake up every morning, after I say my prayers, is "Where am I running today?"'

Jon Sutherland's 3-mile run one Tuesday morning in May 2014 was a very ordinary run in many ways. But in one significant way, it was truly extraordinary. With that run, Sutherland set a new American record for running every single day, the latest run in an unbroken streak going back to 26 May 1969.

With that run, Sutherland extended his running streak to 45 years and two days, passing the record set by his friend Mark Covert, who started his own streak in 1968. Covert's streak ended in 2013 at 16,437 days when he finally gave in to a congenital foot problem and took up cycling instead. Back in the late 60s, the two were teammates at Los Angeles Valley College. They remain close friends. In fact, it was Covert who encouraged Sutherland to keep going and so beat his own record, as authenticated by the US Running Streak Association.

> *Mark told me he had run every day for a year. I go, 'I'm going to try that.' It meant nothing. I did it, I got my year in, no big deal. Pretty soon it's five, 10, 15 years. Now it's 45 years.*

Sutherland, 63 at the time he set the new record, set himself a daily minimum of a mile, but in fact averages more than 11 miles a day, logging more than 190,000 miles in all – with every run documented in detail in 46 binders at his home in West Hills, California.

Sutherland admits there were times when his unbroken run was definitely under threat, not least when he had arthroscopic surgery on both knees. He got round it by running in the morning before he went under the knife – and then running the next afternoon, something he confesses he didn't mention to his surgeon.

Sutherland's first run in the streak came almost two months before Neil Armstrong walked on the moon. In the years that followed, he ran through a rapidly changing world. Making his streak all the more impressive is the fact that for many years Sutherland covered heavy metal bands for music magazines – a job which didn't naturally go hand in hand with running. Employed in the music business variously as a writer, an editor and a publisher, he also managed bands and worked for record labels. And yet, whatever the demands, however anti-social the hours, he always maintained his streak. At one point, he ran 100 miles or more a week for 11 years on the trot.

> *I love it. People, they know that. I mean, that's who I am. If you say, 'Who's Jon Sutherland?' He's a runner. They don't see a rock journo from the 80s. No, he's a runner.*

Inevitably when he was asked when he might stop, it was rock which helped provide his answer. Sutherland quoted the response Metallica's James Hetfield gave when posed the same question: 'I don't see any f***ing stop sign.'

And, as I write, Sutherland is still going strong.

The longest unbroken running streaks

Mark Covert leads the Official USA Retired Running Streak List. The leaders of the Official USA Active Running Streak List (as of 1 April 2016) are:

The Coverts (45+ Years)

Rank, name	Streak start date	City, state, occupation, age	Streak days
1. Jon Sutherland	26 May 1969	West Hills, California, writer, 65	17,113 days (46.85 years)
2. Jim Pearson	16 February 1970	Marysville, Washington, retired, 71	16,847 days (46.12 years)

The Legends (40+ Years)

Rank, name	Streak start date	City, state, occupation, age	Streak days
3. Stephen W. DeBoer	7 June 1971	Rochester, Minnesota, dietician, 60	16,371 days (44.82 years)
4. Alex T. Galbraith	22 December 1971	Houston, Texas, attorney, 65	16,173 days (44.28 years)
5. David L. Hamilton	14 August 1972	Vancouver, Washington, sales, 61	15,937 days (43.63 years)

6. Steven Gathje	25 September 1972	South Minneapolis, Minnesota, actuary, 60	15,895 days (43.52 years)
7. Richard Westbrook	29 December 1973	Jonesboro, Georgia, teacher, 68	15,435 days (42.26 years)
8. Robert R. Kraft	1 January 1975	Miami Beach, Florida, songwriter, 65	15,067 days (41.25 years)
9. James Behr	19 March 1975	Trinity, Florida, educator, 68	14,990 days (41.04 years)

Rick Worley – Something for the weekend!

'If you can run a marathon, you can run life.'

For three years, there probably wasn't much point asking Rick Worley what he was up to that weekend. The Texan runner was busy earning his place in the record books – the Guinness World Record for the most marathons run on consecutive weekends. He clocked up 200 in 159 weeks from 1997 to 2000.

An accomplished businessman, Worley (1947–2010) was the founder of various companies over the years, working in the oil business before retiring to his ranch. His passions were teaching and mentoring, particularly little league baseball.

He also loved to run. 'I probably will never stop,' he announced in 2004. He started running simply to lose weight, but running soon found its own momentum as the marathons took over. Initially his aim was to run his tenth marathon when he turned 40 and then another one when he reached 50 and one more at 60, but when he heard about a runner who finished 50 marathons in the year he turned 50, Worley decided to aim bigger, and so his unbroken weekend run began. Noticing other runners in their 50 States Marathon Club T-shirts, Worley resolved to run every state and the District of Columbia.

But it wasn't just about the marathons for running's sake. Worley added altruism into the mix when he set up a college scholarship fund at Cal Farley's Boys Ranch and Affiliates, near Amarillo. Worley had grown up nearby. As a child, he used to wrestle boys from the home and retained a lasting fondness for all it stood for, particularly its aim to give youngsters a second chance of success in life. He decided the ranch would be the beneficiary of his running as he clocked up the marathons.

However, as 1997 came to an end, Worley still didn't feel he had done enough. He opted to carry on. As he told the *Washington Post*:

> *When the year ended in 97, I had run every weekend. I had run all 50 states and DC. I had finished 59 marathons for the year, but my fundraising hadn't contributed as much as I wanted. Then several people said, 'You know, Rick, if you're wanting to raise more funds, the existing record for the most consecutive weeks to run a marathon is 74. You're already at 59, so why don't you try and break that and see if that doesn't add to the contribution?'*

Worley broke the record for the most successive weekend marathons in June 1998 and celebrated by carrying on. He kept up his run of weekend marathons throughout the rest of the year and then throughout the whole of 1999 as well, adding Canadian provinces and territories and Mexico to his list of conquered lands.

But eventually, everything has to come to an end. Worley announced his streak would end at the Methodist Health Care Houston Marathon on 16 January 2000, the two hundredth marathon in his one hundred and fifty-ninth consecutive week of running weekend marathons. Four teenagers from Cal Farley's Boys Ranch and Affiliates were there to run the race with him. For Worley, their presence kept things in perspective:

> *My streak when it ends is only important if everyone remembers another streak, one that began in 1939. The Boys Ranch will still be here after my running streak ends.*

Worley's reward was his first weekend at his Kingwood, Texas home since the last weekend of December 1996 – and a chance to finish decorating the guest room, a job he'd begun three years before. He died in 2010, but his memory lives on in the Texas Marathon which he started in the year 2000.

David and Linda Major – A marathon couple

*'We aim to inspire the
sedentary general public.'*

David and Linda Major prove there's no need for anyone to become a marathon widow or widower stuck at home. They hold the current Guinness World Record for the most marathons completed by a married couple.

And all from the most unpromising of starts.

David was diagnosed with asthma at the age of two and missed large parts of his early schooling through ill health. He admits that at the age of 29, he was an overweight, unfit, chesty smoker with no energy or motivation to look after himself and was spiralling downwards rapidly. David knew something had to change, and so he started running in 1994.

Linda was born with a hole in her heart. As a child, she was overweight and stood out at school. Her confidence was damaged by bullying. She and David got together as a couple in 1998, and through David's encouragement, she started running in 1999.

The pair, who live near Northampton, have now completed a combined total of more than a thousand marathons. They married on 25 March 2004, the point at which their marathons started counting towards their record. Their first marathon as husband and wife was the Bungay Black Dog Marathon in Suffolk on 4 April 2004. In 2009, they ran a total of 111 marathons between them in one calendar year and became the first married couple in the Marathon Maniacs membership both to achieve ten-star status, an accolade determined on marathon frequency. The last marathon they ran together was the Gran Canaria Marathon on 20 January 2013 in Las Palmas, Spain. David ran 451 marathons in this period of just under 9 years and Linda ran 300. The *Guinness Book of Records* confirmed their world record when it verified their total as 751 marathons.

As well as running for fitness improvement and wanting to feel better about their advancing ages, an important part of their work is in mentoring and encouraging others, from colleagues and friends to complete strangers who think they can't run or don't know how.

> *On our travels, we go out of our way to actively encourage runners to participate more and in turn improve their level of fitness. More importantly, we aim to inspire the sedentary general public who have been looking for a reason to start regular exercise but fear that it is not for 'people like them'.*

Jen Correa – Running back to normality

'Putting it all behind me, as a sign of resilience.'

American fitness site *Daily Burn* declared Jen Correa to be one of the '20 most inspiring runners in the US'. Thirty-seven-year-old Correa was one of the many thousands of people caught up in the devastating Hurricane Sandy, which forced the cancellation of the 2012 New York City Marathon.

Sandy, unofficially known as Superstorm Sandy, hit the States on 29 October and started to claw its way up the eastern seaboard. The government responded with an evacuation order, which included Correa's Oakwood Beach neighbourhood, alongside all low-lying areas of New York and New Jersey.

Correa told the health and fitness magazine *Experience Life* in October 2013:

> *So I loaded up my son, daughter, and nine-year-old shih-tzu and headed*

> *to Brooklyn, where a close friend was letting us stay with her in an inland neighbourhood. Little did I know that the next time I'd see my own house it would be submerged offshore, lost to us forever.*

Correa's husband Peter, an Iraq war veteran, stayed behind to salvage what he could. He was lucky to escape with his life. When the storm struck, he had to swim out of the house and grab onto pieces of debris to reach dry land. 'It's all gone,' was the devastating news he delivered. The water rose to nearly 16 feet. The house floated almost a mile into the weeds and then dropped into the water.

Correa, who writes a blog called *Mom's Gotta Run*, recalls the desperate times:

> *The next day, using a rowboat that had washed inland, we went to our house to see if we could salvage anything. I was able to get my wedding dress and our kids' baptism outfits from the top of my closet, but that was about it. We had lived there for six years and suddenly everything was gone.*

Fortunately, one of the few things the storm couldn't take was Correa's running. Running had always been her sanity, the one thing she did purely for herself. Just the weekend before, she had run 20 miles in preparation for the upcoming New York City Marathon. When it was cancelled, she felt relief, but also a sense that part of her life had gone. Three weeks later, she found the strength to run again.

> *The minute I started running, I realised that I'd come back to my safe place. I didn't have to answer any questions or listen while someone told me how sorry she was for what I was going through. It was just me again. I was choking back the tears. Suddenly I knew I could cry and that it was OK.*

It was the signal Correa needed to start taking care of herself again. Running and surviving had become intertwined. Sandy had destroyed the places she most loved to run, but running itself helped her find another way. Taking inspiration from a cartoon fish in the film *Finding Nemo*, she declares her mantra is 'just keep swimming' – and she did so, running the 2013 NYC Marathon instead, a year later.

Inevitably, the first anniversary of Sandy brought back endless, awful memories, but Correa found strength in the training as the big day approached. For many she symbolised the process of rebuilding thousands of people had to go through. On the NYC Marathon website, they had a tab entitled '26.2 Stories of Hope'. Correa was one of them.

She told Every Mother Counts, a non-profit organisation dedicated to making pregnancy and childbirth safe for every mother:

> *In my heart I'm running for someone else. I received so much help when I needed it, and I'm doing this for everybody out there that needs help. It sounds cheesy, but the truth is there is a time to give and a time to take, in whatever order that presents in*

your life. Some people really need to be given to. Other people start with a whole lot, but then lose it. That's a cycle. I now know both sides of that. I'm a working middle-class person. We owned a home and two cars and occasionally went on vacation. Then, within one day, we were homeless and shopping in a food bank. Nothing is guaranteed. If I can be doing something to help someone else, I'm happy.

Runners undeterred by race cancellation

In the aftermath of Hurricane Sandy, 'will they, won't they' was one of the talking points as pressure mounted both to run the 2012 New York City Marathon and to cancel it. A few people argued it would be a symbol of New York City's strength in adversity; but rather more people argued it would be entirely inappropriate while bodies were still being fished out of the waters.

New Yorker Lauren Mandel was among those having second thoughts about running in the race. Just four days after Superstorm Sandy hit her city, she felt awful as she got closer to the convention centre serving as the hub for race participants. 'Walking past generators heating up tents for people to eat pasta tomorrow night when there are people who haven't eaten a hot meal in five days [left her with the feeling] this is so inappropriate and this is so wrong,' she told news channel CNN.

On the Wednesday, Mayor Michael Bloomberg announced Sunday's race would go ahead as scheduled, but the protests continued to grow, prompting a massive social media backlash, with many calling for a boycott. On the Friday, city and race officials bowed to the pressure, announcing they would cancel the race for the first time in its 42-year history.

The mayor issued a statement:

While holding the race would not require diverting resources from the recovery effort, it is clear that it has become the source of controversy and division.

A key factor was that the starting line was on Staten Island, one of the areas hardest hit by Sandy.

However, an unofficial run was organised on Facebook on the Saturday afternoon by a couple of friends who had spent months fundraising for research into amyotrophic lateral sclerosis – or motor neurone disease, as we would call it in the UK. In the absence of the main New York City Marathon, they decided to race wholly within Central Park, using the example of the original NYC marathon route back in the 1970s. Thirty-five hours later, the Run Anyway New York City Marathon had amassed 1,700 fans on Facebook. On the day, nearly 2,000 runners took part.

CHAPTER FIVE
THE LEGENDS OF MEN'S DISTANCE RUNNING

Emil Zátopek – A unique triple Olympic win

'There is not, and never was, a greater
man than Emil Zátopek.'
AUSTRALIAN ATHLETE RON CLARKE

A statue of Emil Zátopek stands in the grounds of the Olympic Museum in Lausanne, Switzerland. He is the only athlete to be so honoured – recognition of an athlete who dominated like no other. Zátopek (1922–2000) is the only runner to win the 5,000 m, the 10,000 m and the marathon at the same Olympic Games – and all with a style which looked so unpromising.

The *New York Herald Tribune* famously described him: 'bobbing, weaving, staggering, gyrating, clutching his torso, slinging supplicating glances toward the heavens, he ran like a man with a noose around his neck. He seemed on the verge of strangulation.' Zátopek panted and wheezed so much he was nicknamed 'the Locomotive'. He would look utterly exhausted, and yet still he would win.

In the 10,000 m final at the 1948 London Olympics, Zátopek lapped all but two runners and won by more than 300 m to take gold. Three days later, in the final of the 5,000 m, he was 50 m behind at the start of the final lap. A sprint finish all but closed the gap, but he had to be content with silver, just 1.5 m behind the winner.

Four years later in Helsinki, his moment came. The 29-year-old Czech made history. Zátopek won the 10,000 m, took the 5,000 m title and then stepped up to the marathon even though he had never run one before. He won it by two and a half minutes. The *Guardian* reported he crossed the line looking 'like a man who has had a brisk country walk'.

Zátopek's marathon winning time of 2:23:02 was his third world record of the Games in just over a week. Adding extra sparkle to it all was the fact that his wife, Dana Zátopkova, won the javelin event just minutes after Zátopek won the 5,000 m final.

The closest anyone has come to repeating Zátopek's feat was when Finnish athlete Lasse Virén won the 5,000 m and 10,000 m double at the 1976 Montreal Olympics and finished fifth in the marathon. These days, competing in the Olympics' three longest running events in just a week would be unthinkable. However, Zátopek was unstoppable. Between 1949 and 1951 Zátopek took part in 69 long-distance races and won every single one. Over 10,000 m he went undefeated in his first 38 races from 1948 to 1954.

Behind it all, not surprisingly, was exceptionally rigorous training. Zátopek would wear army boots to run in the winter snow and add weights for extra resistance, claiming that it was at the borders of pain and suffering that the men are separated from the boys.

Zátopek later said:

> *There is a great advantage in training under unfavourable conditions. It is better to train under bad conditions, for the difference is then a tremendous relief in a race.*

In an interview with CNN in 2012, his wife, Zátopkova, put his determination down to his upbringing:

> *He had a hard youth. He was working for the Bata shoe company and it was really hard, their training. And their philosophy was 'When there is a barrier don't go around it, go over it'. So this is the philosophy which characterises Emil Zátopek – hard work and when you have a goal, solve it, do it.*

Significantly, Zátopek developed a training regime based on longer runs and shorter, quicker ones. The sport was refining itself all the time.

He explained:

> *Running is easily understandable: you must be fast enough and you must have enough endurance. So*

> *you run fast for speed and repeat it many times*
> *for endurance.*

It was typical of Zátopek that for his first international race in Berlin in 1946, he cycled there from Prague and still managed to win.

After retirement, Zátopek was an outspoken supporter of the Prague Spring temporary liberalisation under Alexander Dubček in 1968. Soviet tanks crushed the uprising in the end, but with the 1968 Mexico Olympics taking place in October that year, the authorities didn't dare be too openly harsh on their dissenting Olympic hero. Zátopek was in the media spotlight. The Soviets chose instead to wait. They later stripped him of his position as a colonel in the Czech army.

His wife, Zátopkova, recalled:

> *Right around the Olympics he was a national hero. It was not possible for the government to punish him. But later during the Soviet occupation he was working as a dustbin man. He got his punishment.*

Zátopek was forced to eke out his living in all manner of menial and dangerous jobs, including well-digging and working in a uranium mine. After the fall of communism in 1989, happier times for the country brought happier times for Zátopek. On 9 March 1990, he was rehabilitated by Václav Havel, the last president of Czechoslovakia and the first president of the Czech Republic. Zátopek's funeral in 2000 saw him honoured by sport's leading figures.

Emil Zátopek's Olympic medals

Helsinki 1952	Marathon	Gold, 2:23:03.2
Helsinki 1952	10,000 m	Gold, 29:17.0
Helsinki 1952	5,000 m	Gold, 14:06.6
London 1948	10,000 m	Gold, 29:59.6
London 1948	5,000 m	Silver, 14:17.8

Jim Peters – Disaster after run of record-breaking marathons

'I was lucky not to have died that day.'

Four times in the 1950s, Jim Peters reduced the record for the world's fastest marathon. In fact, it was Peters who was the first to take the men's marathon under the 2 hour 20 minute mark. And yet today he is probably best remembered as the runner who entered the stadium at the Empire Games marathon with a lead of 17 minutes and yet still failed to finish. The line was in sight, but Peters didn't make it. There is Movietone News footage of his non-finish on YouTube; it's a heart-breaking watch – the sight of a man in utter extremis, at the very limit of his endurance.

I set off too fast in the heat, but that was always my way: to destroy the field... If someone had told me I was

> *so far ahead, I dare say I'd have eased off a*
> *bit... When I woke up in hospital I thought I'd*
> *won. When I asked a nurse, she'd said, 'You*
> *did great, Jim, just great,' so at least I went*
> *back to sleep a winner, didn't I?*

Born in east London, but raised in Becontree in Essex, Peters (1918–1999) was a decent sportsman in his early years. During the war he served in the Royal Army Medical Corps. After the war and by now a qualified optician, he resumed his running, but when he finished only ninth in the 10,000 m at the 1948 Olympics in London, he considered retiring. However, his coach urged him to take up marathon running instead, and it was here that Peters truly made his mark.

When he began, the marathon world record was either 2:26:42 by Japan's Son Kitei in 1935 or a disputed 2:25:39 by Korea's Suh Yun-bok over a course which may have been short in 1947. Peters smashed both, running a new world record of 2:20:42.2 on 14 June 1952 in the Polytechnic Marathon from Windsor to Chiswick. The following year, Peters returned to the course to set a new standard with 2:18:40.4 on 13 June 1953, a record he broke again when he ran 2:18:34.8 that October in the Turku Marathon. He was back at the Polytechnic Marathon the following year to set his fourth and final world marathon record, 2:17:39.4 on 26 June 1954.

When the question of the greatest ever long-distance runner comes up, Peters will always get the most honourable of mentions as the man who single-handedly took the marathon record from 2 hours 25 minutes down to 2 hours 17 minutes, doing so on the back of new speed and strength techniques which also rewrote the training book.

However, his fall was spectacular in Vancouver on 7 August 1954 at the Empire Games, precursor to the Commonwealth Games, on a day so hot the tarmac was melting. Competing in the marathon, Peters entered the sun-drenched stadium with a massive lead in hand and just the last 385 yards around the track to go. His tragedy was that he arrived in a sunstroked state of distress and dehydration – and travelled just 200 m in the next 11 minutes. Peters fell more than half a dozen times and even crawled on all fours at one point. The officials knew they had to hold back, within the bounds of safety. They knew to help him would be to disqualify him. But eventually even the heroic Peters could go no further.

The distinguished journalist Frank Keating recalled the awful spectacle in the *Guardian* in 2007:

> *Instinct and a misbegotten willpower under the merciless sun had Peters keeling over onto the cinder track again and again like a drunken vaudeville tumbler; each time he hauled himself up once more to stagger on in a groggy, futile nobility. When some from the grandstands, unable to bear it, began to shout for a stop, the stadium announcer crassly called for order and 'a respect for sportsmanship'. The ghastly, ghostly mime lasted all of 11 minutes and 200 metres, when a boxer's sprawl of surrender at the halfway mark had the England team's masseur Mick Mayes stepping in to call for stretcher-bearers. Peters, skin a deathly mottled grey and a collar of foam streaming from his mouth, was borne away on a stretcher.*

Peters spent the next 7 hours in an oxygen tent. Of the day itself, he later admitted he couldn't remember a single thing. He never ran again. Arguably, he never fully recovered from his Vancouver trauma, though he lived for many years afterwards. Peters died on 9 January 1999 after a long battle with cancer.

The irony is that Peters was quite possibly robbed of victory. Some say the course was too long. Peters certainly believed so, having apparently measured the course beforehand. The debate continues, but either way, the sympathy was certainly with Peters. That Christmas, the Duke of Edinburgh awarded him an honorary gold medal inscribed 'J. Peters, a most gallant marathon runner', which Peters later described as 'the most treasured of all my trophies'.

Kip Keino – Paving the way

'You come with nothing and you leave with nothing.'

Middle and long-distance running is dominated by East Africans these days. Kip Keino was one of the first to set the pace – not the first Kenyan to win Empire Games or Olympic medals, but certainly the first Kenyan to have a major impact on athletics at an international level.

Born in 1940 in Kenya's Nandi Hills, Keino emerged as a leading distance runner in the mid-1960s, establishing new world records in the 3,000 m (7 minutes 39.6 seconds) and the 5,000 m (13 minutes 24.2 seconds). In his career, he won three Commonwealth gold medals and one bronze – a precursor to the Kenyan runners now at the forefront of world racing.

Perhaps Keino's most famous gold, however, was the gold he won in the 1968 Olympics in Mexico – a trophy earned despite severe abdominal pains, later diagnosed as gallbladder problems. Doctors warned him not to take part, but ignoring their advice, Keino competed in six distance races in eight days. In his first final, the 10,000 m, the pain was so intense he collapsed on the infield with just two laps to go.

> *I had been checked by doctors and found to be suffering from gallstones, but I insisted that I had to take part in the race. I told them that I came to run and I had to because I was representing my country.*

On the day of the 1,500 m final, Keino stayed in bed until about an hour before the race. He then got up, grabbed his kit and boarded a bus, determined to take part. When the bus became stuck in traffic, Kip, already late, jumped off and ran the last 2 miles to the stadium, just in time to register for the race where he faced race favourite, Jim Ryun of the United States. The odds were against him, but the odds counted for nothing. Keino won by 20 m.

He went on to win four Olympic medals in all, also taking silver in the 5,000 m in the Mexico Olympics. At the 1972 Games in Munich, he won silver in the 1,500 m and gold in the 3,000 m steeplechase.

Keino later served as president of Kenya's Olympic committee, but also worked tirelessly for the welfare of his country more generally, taking in more than 100 orphaned children and having seven of his own. His Kipkeino Foundation encompasses the orphanage plus schools and a farm, and also runs an educational programme for the local community, with a special focus on identifying and developing sporting talent.

In 2007, Keino was presented with an honorary Doctor of Laws by the University of Bristol. In the presentation speech, he was praised as:

> One of the greatest athletes of all time; a man who has motivated large numbers of his countrymen to achieve standards in sport which might have been regarded as impossible until he paved the way [...] His creed is 'you come with nothing and you leave with nothing'. One thing is certain: when it is time for Kip to leave, he will leave a great deal, not least many hundreds of young people, all calling him 'Dad'.

Steve Prefontaine – The Muhammad Ali of distance running

'Somebody may beat me, but they are going to have to bleed to do it.'

No one can ever know what Steve Prefontaine would have gone on to achieve; it's a fair bet, though, that it would have been remarkable.

One of the most charismatic runners of his generation, Prefontaine is widely considered one of the greatest American runners of all time. Better known as 'Pre' to the crowds who chanted his name as he ran, he was a runner who captured the imagination, oozing confidence and loving the competition, but also a character, an athlete known for the directness with which he proclaimed his greatness and voiced his determination to be the best.

For Prefontaine, running was an art form:

> *My philosophy is that I'm an artist. I perform an art not with a paint brush or a camera. I perform with bodily movement. Instead of exhibiting my art in a museum or a book or on canvas, I exhibit my art in front of the multitudes.*

Born in Coos Bay, Oregon, in 1951, he discovered his gift for running as a student at Marshfield High School. It was about being the best in the field, but it was also about doing it with style. He combined talent and discipline with star quality. Above all, his running was about expressing something special.

Prefontaine once held the US record in every long-distance event from the 2,000 m to the 10,000 m. In all, he won 119 of the 151 outdoor track races he competed in. 'Even his rare losses were run with flair and determination,' notes USA Track & Field, the national governing body for track and field, long-distance running and race walking in the United States.

> *A lot of people run a race to see who is fastest. I run to see who has the most guts, who can punish himself into exhausting pace, and then at the end, punish himself even more.*

After narrowly missing out on a medal in the 5,000 m in the 1972 Olympics in Munich, Prefontaine was training for the 1976

Montreal Olympics when he was killed in a car crash on 30 May 1975, at the age of 24. Even now, debate continues as to the precise circumstances of his death. No other car was involved.

But no one doubts his influence as a runner who electrified the crowds. Many see him as a key inspiration behind the running boom of the 1970s. In the four decades since, his spirit and his athletic achievements have become the stuff of running legend. Several films have been made documenting his life.

For many, Michael Heald, writer for *Runner's World* magazine, summed it up in a piece in 2013 entitled 'Why Pre Still Matters':

> Pre brought the same urgent swagger to distance running that Muhammad Ali brought to boxing. When Pre talked about running, he made it sound more macho than football, more illuminating than poetry.

Steve Prefontaine is honoured every year at the Prefontaine Memorial Run, a challenging 10k road race across one of his old training courses. Its finish line is at the high school track where he first competed.

Records held by Steve Prefontaine

18 July 1974	2 miles	8:18 (American Record)
8 June 1974	3 miles	12:51 (AR)
26 June 1974	5,000 m	13:21.87 (AR)
27 April 1974	10,000 m	27:43.60 (AR)

Chris Brasher – The man who created the London Marathon

'He did so much for Britain.'
SIR ROGER BANNISTER

On 6 May 1954, Chris Brasher set the pace for a first lap of 57.5 seconds and a second lap of 60.7 seconds in Sir Roger Bannister's successful attempt to break the 4-minute mile on a cinder track in Oxford; two years later, in the 1956 Melbourne Olympics, Brasher finished first in the 3,000 m steeplechase only to be immediately disqualified because of an apparent mid-race collision with the Norwegian Ernst Larsen. Brasher appealed, was found to have done nothing wrong and was eventually awarded gold.

Brasher (1928–2003) went on to become an award-winning journalist and broadcaster, a successful businessman, a racehorse owner, a mountaineer and a conservationist. He served as sports editor of the *Observer* from 1957–1961 and BBC Television's head of general features from 1969–1973. Brasher also built up profitable sportswear and shoe companies and was a pioneer in the sport of orienteering in Britain.

All that would have been enough for one life for most men. But in addition, and above all, Brasher is also the man who founded the London Marathon, a race which remains his greatest legacy.

The idea was hatched on a trip to run the 1979 New York City Marathon. Brasher was hugely taken with what he saw, capturing its flavour in an article he wrote for the *Observer*:

> *Last Sunday, in one of the most trouble-stricken cities in the world, 11,532 men and women from 40*

countries in the world, assisted by over a million black, white and yellow people, laughed and cheered and suffered during the greatest folk festival the world has seen. I wonder whether London could stage such a festival? We have the course, a magnificent course, but do we have the heart and hospitality to welcome the world?

Brasher and his friend and former Melbourne teammate John Disley made sure the answer was yes. Having convinced the police and the various London boroughs the race was both manageable and desirable, they staged the first London Marathon on 28 March 1981. The organisers hoped for 4,000 runners; in fact, more than 7,000 started from Greenwich Park and most of them completed the course.

The 6,255 finishers were led home by the American Dick Beardsley and the Norwegian Inge Simonsen, who staged a spectacular dead heat in the pouring rain on Constitution Hill. Joyce Smith, a 43-year-old mother of two, broke the British record to win the women's race. Among the runners was Brasher himself. At the age of 52, he ran the distance in under 3 hours.

It is worth remembering that the event's success was far from guaranteed. This was before – or perhaps at the start of – the era of the big city marathons. At the time, marathons were generally run in relative anonymity by fitness freaks through the back streets. There was a feeling that marathons simply weren't the domain of ordinary people. Brasher changed all that at a stroke. The inaugural London Marathon was an instant, massive hit, not just with the runners, but also with the spectators who lined the route and with the viewers who watched on television.

Inevitably, the London Marathon quickly expanded. In 1981, there were 20,000 applicants, from which 7,747 runners were selected; a year later, 18,059 were chosen from more than 90,000 applications; before long, it was the biggest marathon in the world, the inspiration for the many marathons which have grown up since.

It is a while since world records have been set on its course, but the London Marathon consistently attracts the cream of world runners, a reflection of its standing and its history as a major event on the world calendar. In all, 962,095 runners completed the London Marathon (1981–2015) in a race shown on television in nearly 200 countries around the world. A record 37,675 people finished in 2015. In April 2016, 39-year-old Shannon Foudy from Hemel Hempstead became the event's millionth finisher.

On his death in 2003, Brasher was lauded for the central role he had played in British athletics for more than 40 years. As the *Guardian* said in its obituary, his race had become 'part of the essence of London'. Writing in the *Daily Mail*, Ian Wooldridge lamented:

> *A great Briton died yesterday morning, leaving our nation a much poorer place. He exemplified the characteristics that built empires without shame, roused thousands of his countrymen and women to get off their backsides and raise millions for the sick and infirm, won an Olympic gold medal, smoked like a chimney, got drunk with me more than twice and, if confronted by the fanatics of political correctness, would have politely requested their absence.*

Men's marathon world records decade by decade

Year	Athlete	Course	Time
1947	Suh Yun-bok (KOR)	Boston	2:25:39
1958	Sergei Popov (URS)	Stockholm	2:15:17
1969	Derek Clayton (AUS)	Antwerp	2:08:33
1988	Belayneh Dinsamo (ETH)	Rotterdam	2:06:50
1999	Khalid Khannouchi (MAR)	Chicago	2:05:42
2008	Haile Gebrselassie (ETH)	Berlin	2:03:59
2014	Dennis Kimetto (KEN)	Berlin	2:02:57

Haile Gebrselassie – World records tumble

'His smile makes athletics smile.'

Jim Denison's 2007 biography of Haile Gebrselassie carries the title *The Greatest*. Few would argue.

Inevitably the Ethiopian's records will be broken, which is precisely the point of records. In fact, it was his own world record that Gebrselassie broke in Berlin in 2008 when he became the first man to run a marathon in under 2 hours 4 minutes. Since then, three other runners have taken the marathon even closer to the great holy grail of the 2-hour mark.

But the measure of a true champion goes beyond results. It's about the way they play the game; and that's why it's likely Gebrselassie's standing will grow with time. Dubbed the 'smiling assassin' for the way he ruthlessly dispatched his competitors on the race course, Gebrselassie will long be remembered as one of the great gentlemen of his sport. 'You were my tailwind and are all record-breaking runners, too!' Gebrselassie said as he set his second successive Berlin world record, running 2:03:59 in 2008 to beat his 2:04:26 of the year before. It seemed typical that he wanted everyone to share in his glory.

> *First, do enough training. Then believe in yourself and say: I can do it. Tomorrow is my day. And then say: the person in front of me, he is just a human being as well; he has two legs, I have two legs, that is all. That is mentally how you prepare.*

While still in his teens Gebrselassie, who was born in Asella, Oromia Region, Ethiopia in 1973, captured a 5,000 m and 10,000 m double at the world junior championships in Seoul, inspired from an early age by the 5,000 m and 10,000 m Olympic double of the great Ethiopian runner Miruts 'The Shifter' Yifter in the 1980 Moscow Games. But it was in 1993 that Gebrselassie really came to prominence: at the age of 20, he won the first of four consecutive world championship titles in the 10,000 m.

Enjoying more than two decades at the top of his profession, he went on to win two Olympic golds. The first was in Atlanta in 1996 over 10,000 m, just beating his rival Paul Tergat. Four years later, in Sydney, he became only the third man in history to retain the title, Tergat again coming second.

Gebrselassie won the Berlin Marathon four times in a row from 2006–2009. Elsewhere, he broke 61 Ethiopian national records and established a succession of new world records, including the 5,000 m, the fastest 10-mile run and the longest distance competed in 1 hour (13 miles 397 yards). 'Haile, Haile,' was the chant from the crowd as he unleashed his trademark blistering finish.

Looking back, Gebrselassie rated his 5,000 m performance at the Weltklasse meeting in Zurich in 1995 as his 'most memorable achievement'. He smashed Moses Kiptanui's record by nearly 11 seconds with a time of 12 minutes 44.39 seconds.

> *You need three things to win: discipline, hard work and, before everything maybe, commitment. No one will make it without those three. Sport teaches you that.*

Gebrselassie announced he was retiring after dropping out of the 2010 New York City Marathon after 25 km. A packed press conference fell silent in disbelief. A week later, there was relief all round when he decided he had been too hasty, far too emotional in the immediate aftermath of disappointment. His results soon vindicated his rethink. After turning 40 in 2013, Gebrselassie set masters (40+) world records for 10 k (28 minutes), 10 miles (47 minutes) and the half-marathon (1:01:09).

The real retirement came in May 2015 at the age of 42. After finishing sixteenth in the Great Manchester Run, he called time on a 25-year career which had brought him eight World Championship victories and seen him set 27 world records in total.

His manager, Jos Hermens, seemed to sum up his career perfectly: 'His smile makes athletics smile.' But even as he retired, Gebrselassie made it clear he had no intention to stop running altogether. He told the BBC: 'I'm retiring from competitive running, not from running. You cannot stop running. This is my life.'

Away from competing, Gebrselassie had always been one of his sport's great ambassadors including work as a mentor for G4S 4teen, a programme supporting 14 young athletes from 13 countries ahead of the 2012 London Olympics. He is also a successful businessman in his own right back home in Ethiopia where he employs more than 1,000 people, works in real estate projects and owns four hotels and a coffee plantation.

Haile Gebrselassie's personal outdoor bests

6 June 1999	1,500 m	Stuttgart	3:33.73
27 June 1999	1 mile	Gateshead	3:52.39
22 August 1997	2,000 m	Brussels	4:56.1
28 August 1998	3,000 m	Brussels	7:25.09
31 May 1997	2 miles	Hengelo	8:01.08
13 June 1998	5,000 m	Helsinki	12:39.36
1 June 1998	10,000 m	Hengelo	26:22.75

11 December 2002	10 km	Doha	27:02
11 November 2001	15 km	Nijmegen	41:38
27 June 2007	20,000 m	Ostrava	56:25:98
15 January 2006	20 km	Phoenix	55:48
27 June 2007	1 hour	Ostrava	21,285 m
15 January 2006	Half-marathon	Phoenix	58:55
12 March 2006	25 km	Alphen aan den Rijn	1:11:37
20 September 2009	30 km	Berlin	1:27:49
28 September 2008	Marathon	Berlin	2:03:59

Paul Tergat – No more Mr Silver

'At last! Some people said, "You cannot win a race," but I knew my day would come. I knew nothing was going to stop me.'

It seemed that Paul Tergat was in danger of being the perennial Mr Silver – until a magnificent day in Berlin in 2003.

With five straight world cross-country titles to his credit, Tergat's credentials weren't in doubt, but the Kenyan struggled to transfer his cross-country dominance to track and road where a frustrating second place invariably seemed to be his lot in the important races. Tergat seemed fated to remain in Haile Gebrselassie's shadow. He finished as runner-up to the Ethiopian in the 10,000 m in the Olympics in 1996 in Atlanta; in Sydney, in 2000, he was second to Gebrselassie by an agonising nine-hundredths of a second. He was also second in the 1997 and 1999 World Championships.

As for marathons, Tergat, born in 1969 in Kabarnet, Baringo, Kenya, just wasn't winning them either. Doubt was setting in. There was a feeling that at 181 cm (5 feet 11 and a half inches), he just wasn't compact enough to be a world-record marathoner. But all that began to change in 2003. From his marathon in London that spring, he said he knew he could become the first man to break the 2-hour 5-minute barrier. Berlin then became his exclusive focus throughout the summer; 'mission world record', as he called it. All his efforts paid off gloriously.

> *I always said I know that my time in the marathon will come if I stay focused. And I felt that I would be able to break the marathon one day. Now that has happened, and I am very happy.*

On 28 September 2003, Tergat not only won in the German capital, but set a new world men's marathon record, the first Kenyan to do so. Fellow Kenyans Tegla Loroupe and Catherine Ndereba had held the world record in the women's marathon; but until Tergat, no Kenyan man had been the fastest marathoner in the world.

Berlin was Tergat's sixth marathon and his first victory. The 34-year-old ran 42.2 km (26.2 miles) in 2:04:55, shattering by 43 seconds the previous record held by the Moroccan-born American

Khalid Khannouchi, set in London in 2002. And he might have done even better had it not been for a little confusion going through the Brandenburg Gate, just before the finish. Tergat lost several seconds trying to figure out which of the towering pillars he was supposed to run through. 'There was nobody there to show me,' he explained later.

Thereafter it was a thrilling sprint finish as Tergat battled with his pacemaker and fellow Kenyan Sammy Korir. Tergat prevailed. Korir finished just 1 second behind him, also smashing Khannouchi's previous benchmark.

> I knew deep in my head one day I will get the world record. I told all my friends my time would come, despite some of them saying I was too tall. [...] The marathon is a matter of experience. After five attempts, today was a completely different perspective.

Tergat's focus these days is his Paul Tergat Foundation, which works to 'mobilise resources to promote the well-being of mankind'. Its particular emphasis is to work with disadvantaged and marginalised people and communities, creating sustainable programmes to promote access to food, education, health and other basic human needs. The emphasis is on creating 'vibrant, healthy, informed and economically empowered African communities' and, in doing so, nurturing 'that great potential which exists in rural communities in Africa'.

Paul Tergat's career highlights

2003	Berlin Marathon	2:04:55 (World record)
2001 and 2002	London Marathon	2nd
2001	Chicago Marathon	2nd
2000	Sydney Olympics, 10,000 m	Silver
1999 and 2000	World Half-marathon	Champion
2000	Lisbon, Portugal half-marathon	59:05 (WR)
1997	Brussels, 10,000 m	26:27.85 (WR)
1997 and 1999	World Championships, 10,000 m	Silver
1996	Atlanta Olympics, 10,000 m	Silver
1995	World Championships, 10,000 m	Bronze
1995–1999	World Cross-country	Five-time champion

CHAPTER SIX

DEFEATING THE TERRORISTS

Theresa Giammona – Honouring a beloved husband

*'I never thought these would be the last
words that I would say to my husband.'*

New York firefighter Vincent Giammona was on the verge of fulfilling a long-held ambition. He was turning 40 on 11 September 2001, and in February that year, he secured the perfect way to celebrate it, a place in the New York City Marathon that November.

As his wife, Theresa, recalls, running was central to Vinny's life. He was a family man, a devoted husband and a doting father to their four children. But he was also a man who loved to run:

> *Vinny was a runner his whole life. It was a huge part of his daily fitness routine. He would go for a run and our daughter, Frankie, would follow her dad on her bicycle as he ran.*

Theresa had arranged a family treat for Vinny's fortieth birthday on that fateful September day. Vinny had worked a 24-hour shift and stayed at the station on the morning of 11 September to go for a birthday run. Theresa spoke to him on the phone to plan their day.

But then the world changed. Terrorists attacked New York's landmark twin towers. A friend phoned Theresa to tell her what had happened; Theresa phoned Vinny at the fire station. She spoke to him just as he was setting out for the World Trade Center with his fellow firefighters from Engine 24 and Ladder 5.

> *He was off duty and responded as a volunteer. I told him to be careful and never thought these would be the last words that I would say to my husband. On 11 September 2001, my husband, Lt Vincent Giammona, made the supreme sacrifice along with 342 FDNY (Fire Department City of New York) brothers, 37 PAPD (Port Authority Police Department) officers and 23 NYPD (New York City Police Department) officers.*

Just a few weeks later, on Sunday, 4 November 2001, friends, fellow firefighters and Vinny's sister combined for the perfect tribute: they raced the New York City Marathon for him, in his memory, combining as a relay team. Eight years later, in 2009,

Vinny's younger brother, Steven, ran the NYC marathon in Vinny's trainers in Vinny's honour. In 2015, Theresa followed suit, running the marathon for the charity which had seen her through, the New York Police and Fire Widows' and Children's Benefit Fund.

Theresa comfortably sailed past her fundraising target of $3,600, eventually reaching $6,871. As for the race, she finished in 5:40:21. She felt Vinny was with her every step of the way. She told *Runner's World*:

> Time does heal, but you never forget, you know? Vinny and I were only married nine years, and we were blessed with four beautiful kids. We didn't even make it to our ten-year anniversary. But if you told me back then 'You're only going to get this amount of time,' I would do it all over again.

Kevin Parks – Building a network of support

'How the country – and the world – reacted to this is a testament to how strong it is.'

Kevin Parks was celebrating his run in the Boston Marathon on 15 April 2013 when, just six blocks away, terrorists detonated two pressure-cooker bombs at the finish line near the city's Copley Square. Parks turned to his best friend sitting beside him – the same friend he had turned to 12 years earlier at school when he heard the news of the 9/11 atrocities, attacks which killed his father, Bob, a bond broker on Wall Street.

Parks' response wasn't anger on that April day in Boston. Instead, he felt comfort that he was surrounded by people he loved. He also felt renewed determination to channel his own grief into helping others. As he told the *Huffington Post*:

> *If there is any silver lining, it is the unbelievable support you receive from people in times like that. That is a similar thing that happened after Boston. How the country – and the world – reacted to this is a testament to how strong it is.*

For Parks, commemoration of his own father is enshrined in his work for Tuesday's Children, a body founded to promote long-term healing among all those directly affected by the events of Tuesday, 11 September 2001. Its mission today is to keep the promise to those children and families, though these days the remit goes beyond the attack on the Twin Towers. The charity aims to serve and support communities affected by acts of terror worldwide.

Very much one of Tuesday's children himself, Parks, now an investment analyst in midtown Manhattan, is one of the charity's most fervent supporters. On 1 November 2015, for the sixth successive year, he ran the New York City Marathon on the charity's behalf.

Parks began the marathon knowing his five previous fundraising campaigns had raised nearly $150,000. In 2014 alone, his donation was around $75,000.

It is only in recent years, however, that Parks has spoken about his loss. His father worked in One World Trade Center at Cantor

Fitzgerald, which lost 658 of its 960 New York employees that day. Final confirmation of his death didn't come until two weeks later.

> The message [our neighbour] sort of gave us, and it's hard to think of it this way, was that they said we were lucky we found his body. So we were comforted by that and to have some level of closure.

As part of Tuesday's Children's ongoing work, the charity helped build a resiliency centre in Newtown, Connecticut, to provide therapy and healing programmes in the wake of the shooting which killed 20 children and six teachers at Sandy Hook Elementary School on 14 December 2012.

Brian Kelley – The running world unites

> 'We will all be with you as you learn to stand and walk and, yes, run again.'
> BARACK OBAMA

In the aftermath of the Boston Marathon bombing, US President Barack Obama told the city it would run again. It was inevitable that it would. Within minutes of the blasts, social media was abuzz. For many millions, running is about freedom, and it was therefore freedom that was under attack. The natural response was to keep on running.

At an interfaith service in Boston's Cathedral of the Holy Cross just days after the bombing, Obama said:

> *Our prayers are with the injured – so many wounded, some gravely. From their beds, some are surely watching us gather here today. And if you are, know this: as you begin this long journey of recovery, your city is with you. Your commonwealth is with you. Your country is with you. We will all be with you as you learn to stand and walk and, yes, run again. Of that I have no doubt. You will run again. You will run again. Because that's what the people of Boston are made of. Your resolve is the greatest rebuke to whoever committed this heinous act. If they sought to intimidate us, to terrorise us, to shake us from [...] the values that make us who we are, as Americans, well, it should be pretty clear by now that they picked the wrong city to do it.*

Across America and around the world, runs were planned as acts not just of commemoration, but also of solidarity, often under the Boston Strong banner. Runners began to gather. 'It's simple,' said Brian Kelley, who organised the San Francisco gathering. 'This is what we do.' Kelley was at work as a designer at the *San Francisco Chronicle* at the time of the attacks. He had no personal connections with Boston, but the attack felt deeply personal. He felt compelled to take action. He did so through a rallying cry on his popular *Pavement Runner* blog:

> *I feel like I need to do something. Something more than a donation. Something more than a blog post*

*or a photo or a graphic. I'm inspired by the
community and how we have come together
and shown our support, shed our tears and
expressed our fears. With a simple look at
your Facebook page, a refresh of your Twitter
feed or scroll through Instagram, you can
SEE the love. But I want to FEEL it. I want
us to embrace the community in a REAL and
HUMAN way. I want us to do what we do best.
I want us to run... together.*

He called for a 'run for us to unite and show our strength, a run
for those that were unable to finish, a run for those that may never
run again, a run for us to try and make sense of the tragedy that
has forever changed something we love'.

Blogs, Facebook and Twitter were the means by which he rallied
his army of peace for a mass, simultaneous run as far and wide as
possible, on Monday 22 April, a week after the one hundred and
seventeenth Boston Marathon and all its tragedy. As he stressed,
it didn't matter how many ran. All that mattered was that they
did it together. And so it spread. Within six months, more than
121 cities had responded. Elsewhere, John Beatty, a 38-year-
old engineer at NASA's jet propulsion laboratory in Pasadena,
California, was organising his own Unity Runs.

> *In the world of running, there is one
> constant truth: there is always a
> runner out there willing to help you.
> Whether it is to share something that they have
> learned along the way or to simply run next to
> you on a long weekend run or race day, there is*

always someone there. This is what immediately made me fall in love with the sport of running. From my very first marathon to the way the running world came together after the 2013 Boston Marathon, the community will always be there with open arms, myself included.

Juli Windsor – Overcoming disability and terrorist attack

*'Overwhelmed with sadness
and heartbroken for those who
lost loved ones today.'*

On 21 April 2014 3-foot 9-inch Juli Windsor made history as the first runner with dwarfism to complete the Boston Marathon. She was subsequently named by *SELF* magazine as among the 'Most Inspirational Women to Have Ever Run the Boston Marathon' – a just acknowledgment of a triumph of perseverance, on the back of considerable courage.

A physician assistant in Boston with a special interest in adolescent mental health and the health needs of adopted children, Windsor was born with a rare form of dwarfism. Her life has been about using her stature to her advantage as a platform to talk with teenagers about self-acceptance – all the easier for the fact that she can often greet younger people at eye level. As she says on her website, Windsor considers herself a leader who brings to light the beauty of living with differences; someone who likes to challenge social norms and public perceptions.

Early on, Windsor discovered a love of running – something received wisdom suggested she really oughtn't to be doing:

> *For the most part, running is discouraged for people with dwarfism. You have a higher risk of developing osteo-arthritis, and just the pressure that running can have on the joints. It's different for us. It's not an encouraged thing.*

For Windsor, however, it felt natural, and as her love of running deepened, with it soon came the dream of running the Boston Marathon. Taking more than twice the number of steps other runners require, she was on the verge of realising that ambition on 15 April 2013 when the Boston bombers struck. Twenty-seven-year-old Windsor and her friend John Young were looking at a 4 hours 30 minutes finishing time, half a mile from becoming the first dwarfs to complete the course when terrorists struck, killing three people and injuring more than 260.

Windsor and Young finally crossed the line fifteen days later. Still struggling to comprehend what had happened, they sought closure by returning to the point where they were stopped, at Charlesgate and Commonwealth Avenue. They then resumed their run and continued to the finish. Young wore his shirt and number from the race; Windsor wore a shirt proclaiming *Run Your Heart Out Boston*. When they crossed the line, Windsor's husband, Blake, put a medal around her neck; Young's son, Owen, placed the medal around his.

Windsor told the *Boston Globe*:

> *It's a surreal feeling. It brings back the panic, the concern of the unknown, of not knowing what's going on. There's also an exhilaration ... a hope of the feeling of some completeness.*

They both made sure they would be back for 2014 to reclaim their race fully and enjoy the finish they were denied in 2013. Sadly, it wasn't to be for Young who had to withdraw during the race due to illness. But for Windsor the day surpassed expectations, not least for the fact that she found herself at the very head of the race. Windsor was part of the mobility-impaired group which included around 20 athletes with disabilities. At 8:50 a.m., they were the first ones out on the course.

> *For the first 10 miles, I was leading the Boston Marathon. We played it up. Everybody would go, 'Juli Windsor is in the lead.' By about mile 10, the wheelchair athletes caught up, and by mile 13, the elite women caught up. It was so fun to watch them pass by. They just blew me away. The crowds yesterday, you couldn't even imagine. I think there was such a sense of pride and community that was felt. I could take my fist, raise it up and go, 'Boston!' It was so fun to play to the crowd and get a response out of everybody. It was just an incredible race.*

New York runner Danh Trang, 27, who was born with a form of dwarfism known as achondroplasia, also completed the marathon, raising more than $14,000 for Little People of America, an organisation dedicated to improving the quality of life for those with dwarfism. Trang finished in 5:36:48; Windsor secured her place in history with a finish time of 4:43:26.

> *I think that overall we all have this idea that people with disabilities have these challenges to overcome, and that life must be so hard, and that 'my life has to be better than theirs'. But in my perspective this is what my life is, and I want people to see that and understand that this is just a beautiful way of living.*

Lynn Crisci – Survivor turned marathon runner

'You can do anything if you want it badly enough.'

One of the most moving and compelling photographs of the 2014 Boston Marathon shows runner Lynn Crisci in tears as she talks to a reporter after finishing the race. The image caps a remarkable journey for Boston resident Crisci, proof that she could come back not once, but twice.

A rising singer and performer, Crisci fell in a stage accident in 2006 that left her bedridden for three years with severe neck, head and spinal cord injuries, in addition to suffering from the connective tissue disorder Ehlers-Danlos Syndrome and fibromyalgia. She had to learn basic skills all over again. It took her six years to go from wheelchair to walking again; and life was looking up. She was 'especially thrilled' to be walking without a cane and to be reclaiming her career in the arts: 'It was really exciting to get a second chance at life.'

And then terrorists struck at the 2013 Boston Marathon. For Crisci, new wounds reopened the old:

> *I think a lot of survivors see themselves as different now forever, a new person, the me before the marathon is not the me now. A therapist explained it very well. He said everybody else was traumatised; you were retraumatised.*

Crisci, who was among the crowds, recalls the first explosion:

> *I was looking in that direction. That's where the runners were heading. It was all so fast. I just saw fire everywhere. There were people everywhere. It was just such a crowded sidewalk on Marathon Monday. And then suddenly it was just fire everywhere, just in that second. And within two or three more seconds, it was grey to black smoke, and it went up five storeys high, like the whole building in front of you. And within a second after that, the smoke rolled over your head like a wave of water. It just felt that the whole world around you disappeared into that smoke.*

Crisci survived, but at a price, escaping with a painful lower back injury, temporary hearing loss and post-traumatic stress disorder. She describes herself in the weeks that followed as stumbling around, unable to hear, unable to think and feeling as if a wall now divided her and her fellow survivors from the rest of the world that had not experienced the awfulness they had been through. As she began to emerge from it all, she began to realise what she had to do: to complete the Boston Marathon the following year.

Having fought her way out of a wheelchair, she was determined to fight her way across the finishing line too, all in aid of the US Pain Foundation, a non-profit organisation created by people with pain for people with pain.

Focusing on a place at the start line in the mobility-impaired division, Crisci spent five months in rehabilitation, eventually working up to power walking on a treadmill. She also joined 415 Strong, a group of 20 bombing survivors, who ran together every Saturday morning. It worked. In a moment of unimaginable pride and triumph, she crossed the line which a year before had been a scene of horror.

> *I feel like that was definitely one of the proudest moments in my life. No matter how many fears I carried for the rest of my life [...] I can still tell myself 'You can do anything if you want it badly enough and you put your mind to it. You finished the Boston Marathon!'*

But Crisci remains realistic. She knows there is still a long way to go. Nearly two years on, Boston's Copley Square still induces a feeling of panic as she relives the horror of it all; and much of her life is spent shuttling between the ten doctors she sees for the physical and cognitive therapies she needs to deal with her lingering injuries. As of March 2015, in an interview with *USA Today*, she said she still suffered from a frontal-lobe brain injury, hearing impairment, lower-back injury, loud ringing in her ears and severe post-traumatic stress disorder.

But as she says, the marathon was her way of telling herself she was more capable and much stronger than she realised. It was also about giving hope to others.

Georges Salines – The man who kept running

*'She was a great young woman who loved
life passionately. She was also a citizen
of the world, a person of peace.'*

On the evening of Friday, 13 November 2015, a series of coordinated terrorist attacks in Paris left 130 people dead and 368 injured. Among those who perished was Lola Salines, the 28-year-old daughter of Georges Salines, who went on to become the president of the support group which was created amid the shock and misery which followed, the November 13 Association: Fraternity and Truth.

In the awful aftermath of the attacks, Salines, a runner since his student days, admitted that running became even more necessary than ever to his life and well-being. For years, three times a week, on the edge of the Bois de Vincennes, he would slip on his trainers and run for an hour. Following the terrorist attacks, ritual became therapy.

Lola was in the Bataclan theatre on the Friday night where the American rock band Eagles of Death Metal were in the middle of their performance when three gunmen wearing suicide belts forced their way in and started shooting people at random. In its tribute, French newspaper *Le Monde* said it was impossible to find a photograph of Lola in which she wasn't smiling. Eighty-nine people were killed in the theatre alone.

Salines, a 59-year-old doctor, recalled:

> *I learnt she had died on the Saturday around 6 p.m. On the Sunday morning, I had training. I went along to see my friends and to run with them.*

For friends and fellow runners, Salines' run that morning became their way to show their solidarity. More than a hundred runners turned up simply because they knew Salines would be there. Out of respect, some didn't dare speak to him – a gesture Salines appreciated: 'They were all around me. They were extraordinary. It did me good.'

In the weeks that followed, Salines' workload with the support group was immense, including media duties and high-level meetings. But the running didn't stop. He called it his *'fenêtre de respiration'*, his breathing window. He predicted legal cases stretching years ahead and plenty more psychological shocks to come. He was proved tragically right when it was Brussels' turn to fall victim to terrorist attack on the morning of 22 March 2016:

> *It revives the pain, the stress. You think constantly of what the families are going through, the near ones who all day long are trying to get through on a mobile phone which doesn't answer.*

The battle goes on. Running helps him keep it all in perspective. When running with friends, he enjoys the chat; when running alone, his thoughts turn to his daughter, and through those thoughts he reaches what he describes as a state of mind close to meditation. 'Yes, ideas come. These are moments when you are not looking at your mobile, not watching television. These are moments when you think.'

But there is no bitterness, simply the hope that mankind might one day find a solution.

> *We are all human beings. We have all got a head, two arms, two legs. We all live on the same small planet. I don't know what we can do against terrorism, but I think that to find a long-term solution, we have got to break down barriers rather than build up walls.*

In its four decades of existence, the Paris Marathon has only ever been cancelled once — in 1991, during the First Gulf War.

Runners and organisers alike were determined that the fortieth Paris Marathon would go ahead exactly as planned in April 2016, five months after the terror attacks on the French capital. Inevitably, it did so amid hugely increased security, everyone mindful too of the bombings which had rocked the Boston Marathon three years before.

France remained in a state of emergency, imposed after the November attacks, with thousands of armed soldiers and police patrolling the streets. The March 2016 Brussels attacks, just 12 days before the Paris Marathon, heightened tensions further.

Marathon director Edouard Cassignol confirmed:

Safety is a major concern today, and security is the responsibility of the state authorities. We've had regular meetings with police and officials in Paris in recent weeks and we can say that security has been considerably strengthened.

Traffic was restricted in vulnerable areas, electronic surveillance was increased and helicopters were deployed to monitor the event. Additional emergency crews were on hand. Bag searches were increased, as was the number of security guards. Trained staff were on the lookout for any abnormal behaviour, and the race's 3,000 volunteers were briefed on the need for vigilance.

More than 50,000 runners took part on the day, looping from the Champs-Élysées back round to the Arc de Triomphe, via the Bois de Vincennes, the Seine and the Bois de Boulogne. Tens of thousands of spectators lined the streets.

The marathon passed off successfully.

CHAPTER SEVEN
CONQUERING DISABILITY

David Kuhn – The blind runner running to beat cystic fibrosis

'To date, the journey has been nothing less than amazing.'

David Kuhn is a man on a mission, a blind runner determined to run roughly 11,000 miles around the United States to raise money for the Cystic Fibrosis Foundation. His sole concern is to help raise the money to fund the research which might buy extra time for his stricken granddaughter.

Kuhn was 29 years old in 1981 when he started to lose his eyesight following a car crash involving a drunk driver. 'I was not ready for that,' he told the *Bismarck Tribune*. 'My life was changed forever.'

However, his first marathon didn't come until many years later, in 2009. Kuhn was employed as a director at a senior services centre and was looking for fundraising ideas. Running a marathon seemed a good idea, and Kuhn volunteered to run the Chicago Marathon. His problem was that, by then, his eyesight had deteriorated to the extent that he needed to be tethered to another runner. After his first guide fell through, he worried he would be a burden, but when a running colleague spread the news he was looking for a replacement, Kuhn received more than 250 offers within just a few days.

The world was nothing but a blur to him, but Kuhn had found the challenge he was looking for — and he rose to it. He went on to take part in 24 marathons around the US including five Chicago Marathons, three Boston Marathons and the California International Marathon.

> *I have had so many wonderful things happen to me as direct result of losing my eyesight that, if my ophthalmologist told me that if you get here tomorrow I can restore your eyesight, I would tell him no.*

In recent years, Kuhn's running gained particular focus when his granddaughter Kylie was diagnosed with cystic fibrosis, a genetic disease that attacks mostly the lungs, the pancreas, the liver and the intestine. Diagnosis meant Kylie's life would be sadly limited — a fact which inspired Kuhn to go for the big one. In 2014, at the age of 62, he set out to run around the perimeter of the United States. From Seattle, the idea was to head east to Bangor, south to Jacksonville and then turn west to San Diego before turning north to head back to Seattle again, a total of around 11,000 miles. Crucial to his thinking was the fact that the undertaking was wholly his choice.

> *When I consider some of the struggles that Kylie and people with cystic fibrosis [endure], my aches and pains [from the run] are really nothing, because I can quit. I can say tomorrow is it and they can't.*

Kuhn's aim was to raise $500,000 for cystic fibrosis research; his goal was to run at least 20 miles a day either on a track or on a path with the help of sighted runners. As he says, others have the scientific knowledge to fight the disease; he simply had his running. He made the point, as echoed in the title of his blog, *It's All I Can Do* – home to his very direct appeal for support.

But sadly the logistics were against him. With 1,899 miles completed, he couldn't get the support he needed and was forced to put the run on hold. As of September 2015, Kuhn confirmed he was still looking for an organiser to help him. It was all that was holding him back. As soon as he found the support he needed, he pledged he would head straight back to Wisconsin and pick up his run where he left off. Kuhn remains determined to head back out and finish the amazing journey he started in 2014.

Team Hoyt – More than a thousand races together

> *'We haven't figured out what kind of vegetable he is yet.'*

Dick and Judy Hoyt were told that their son Rick had little hope of a normal life when he was born in 1962. Rick was diagnosed as a spastic quadriplegic with cerebral palsy, as a result of oxygen deprivation to his brain at the time of his birth. His parents were advised he would be far better off hidden away – advice they made it their mission to prove utterly wrong.

As Dick told ABC News:

> When Rick was born, they said, 'Forget him. Put him away. Put him in an institution. He's going to be nothing but a vegetable for the rest of his life.' And here he is. He's 52 years old and we haven't figured out what kind of vegetable he is yet.

Rick's parents' vision was that he should be included in the community, in sports, in education and one day in the workplace – a vision they turned into reality. Running has been the means to their end.

Rick couldn't walk or speak, but Dick and Judy realised his eyes would follow them around the room. They realised their first priority was to find a way to help Rick communicate for himself. With $5,000, a group of engineers at Tufts University built an interactive computer for Rick in 1972. Using his head, Rick could highlight selected letters. He had found a voice, and instantly it was obvious he was mad on sport.

Team Hoyt was born in 1977 when Rick told his father he wanted to participate in a 5-mile benefit run for a lacrosse player who had been paralysed in an accident. Dick agreed to push Rick in his wheelchair. That night Rick told his father, 'Dad, when I'm running, it feels like I'm not handicapped.' A one-off race became a way of life. They went on to complete hundreds of races, including marathons, duathlons and triathlons.

The Boston Marathon was always a favourite, a race where they gained fixture status over the years, a Boston institution year after year, always recognisable, Rick in his custom-built racing wheelchair, Dick pushing behind. For many, they embodied the heart and soul of the event.

The 2009 Boston Marathon was officially Team Hoyt's thousandth race, but eventually age began to catch up with Dick. After more than 30 Boston Marathons together and with Dick now 73, they decided Boston 2013 would be their last one together. They decided they would continue to do the shorter races and triathlons together, but they would have to call it a day when it came to the marathons.

However, 2013 was the year of the bombings. Dick and Rick were unable to complete the course. But they were not to be denied their swansong, returning in 2014 to celebrate not just their running partnership, but also to honour the human spirit which had been so much in evidence in the aftermath of the marathon bomb atrocities.

Their final Boston Marathon inevitably became an event in itself. The duo frequently had to stop to acknowledge the crowds before they finally reached the finishing line in 7:37:33, their thirty-second and final Boston Marathon. Fellow runners accompanied them over the line, adjusting their pace to finish with them.

But it wasn't quite the end of an era. Dick stepped back, but Rick resolved to keep going. Friend and supporter Bryan Lyons took over and pushed Rick in the 2015 Boston Marathon. Dick was also there, returning in a rather more vaunted capacity. Recognising his achievement, the Boston Athletic Association invited him back as race grand marshal, an honour that saw him ride ahead of the elite group on race day and then join the mayor, the governor and other dignitaries at the finish.

It's not going to be sad. I'm 75. I really, really love running Boston. To us, it's the best marathon in

the world. My big thing is for Rick to be able
to continue... and there's tons of people who
want to push Rick.

The Schneider twins – Running with autism

'I tearfully cheer and
think of how inspiring they
are to so many.'

New York twins Alex and Jamie Schneider are both severely autistic. They are non-verbal, and they are deemed very challenging in their behaviour. But they have both found the meaning to their lives in running, thanks to the love and support of their parents, Robyn and Allan.

Even now, the memory of that first diagnosis remains vivid for Robyn:

> *It took only a few minutes and one word to change our world forever. 'Autism.' Confusion, shock, sadness and pain quickly transformed us into energised and unrelenting parents, determined to seek the best educational programme and medical treatment for our sons.*

When the boys turned five and with limited help available, Robyn and Allan Schneider became the founding parents at the Eden II Genesis School on Long Island, an intensive behavioural programme solely for children with autism. But the turning point was their discovery of running. The Schneiders contacted the Rolling Thunder Running Club who tested the boys out.

> *It seemed to be an eternity, but 30 minutes later, there they all were, running toward us at full speed. We could see the boys were smiling and overly excited as they approached. That was a pivotal moment for us as a family, as our journey took on a new direction. Gushing with enthusiasm, they told us that Alex and Jamie were 'natural' runners with unlimited potential!*

It was a question of finding the right coach for Alex, the faster of the two. Kevin McDermott stepped in, recognised Alex as a veritable running machine and trained him to a personal best of 3:14:36 in the 2013 New York City Marathon. The twins have gone on to run more than 125 mainstream races in the area and have become celebrities among the running community.

Their disability requires them to run with coaches to direct them through the course, to make sure they rehydrate, to watch out for hazards and to guard against them overheating – all aspects they cannot monitor themselves. Autism also means that they run with greater freedom than other runners: the freedom of never knowing how long each race is. Their approach is running at its simplest: to run as fast as they can until they reach the finishing line. They remain completely dependent and will always require 24-hour supervision; but running now defines them.

Mother Robyn again:

> *Race day is always a special and exciting day for us all. My emotions are high as I wait impatiently at the finish line. I watch first for Alex, and then Jamie. And as they each approach the finish line, my heart pounding rapidly, I tearfully cheer and think of how inspiring they are to so many and how proud I am of their accomplishments.*

It was Alex's speed that saved the family when the bombers struck at the Boston Marathon in 2013. He crossed the line 45 minutes before the first bomb exploded, which meant the family was clear of the grandstands before the mayhem. Jamie hadn't yet approached the finishing line at that point. But that's not to say the brothers were unaffected. Far from it. For Alex and Jamie, 22 years old at the time, the trauma was greater in some ways than it was for those who can verbalise their experiences.

As their father Allan told the *New York Times*:

> *They can't talk it out like you or me could. We can try telling them everything's going to be OK, but they still don't understand what happened. We can't explain what a bomb is. We don't know how they internalize all this stuff.*

Robyn has written a memoir, *Silent Running: Our Family's Journey to the Finish Line with Autism*. She knows that her sons will never be able to read the book, but through it she has left a legacy for them, and has ensured that their story will live on.

Claire Lomas – 'The making of me'

'Claire is a force of nature. Give her a challenge that seems impossible and she will smash it to bits.'
CLARE BALDING

On 6 May 2007, top-level event rider Claire Lomas suffered a devastating horse riding accident during the Osberton horse trials in Nottinghamshire. She fractured her neck, dislocated her back, fractured ribs, punctured a lung and subsequently developed pneumonia. She was left paralysed from the chest down.

For most people, their active life would have stopped right there. However, for Lomas, the trauma wasn't the end of the line. It was a starting point, a stepping stone towards a string of achievements that have made her a familiar and hugely respected figure in disabled athletics.

Lomas discharged herself from hospital after only eight weeks, did lots of rehab and over time found the strength and courage to rebuild her life. A year after her accident she met and later married Dan and had a baby girl, Maisie. Continuing her upward course, Lomas tried new sports including skiing, hand-cycling and motorbikes, set up a business and fundraised to help find a cure for paralysis.

In 2012, Lomas provided us with one of the great images of the bravery and endurance the London Marathon stands for, when she crossed the finishing line 17 days after the starting gun. The first (and only) paralysed person to walk the London Marathon, she did it in a pioneering £43,000 robotic suit, which allowed her to 'walk' by detecting shifts in her balance. Trusting her legs would even take her weight when she had no sensation at all was tough, she said. But she made it, supported and encouraged by husband Dan.

Thirty-two-year-old Lomas raised £210,000 for Spinal Research along the way – reward for the immense effort and concentration which lay behind every single step on a journey that took her into the hearts of the nation. Crossing the line under an arch of red balloons, Lomas declared: 'It's a moment I am going to treasure for the rest of my life.'

She told the BBC from the finishing line:

> *That last half a mile or so was pretty easy to walk because I just had everyone pushing me forward. But it has been very challenging, hard on my arms, very hard mentally because I could not feel my legs and have to concentrate on every step.*

Her achievement made news around the world.

A year later Lomas completed another challenge, hand-cycling 400 miles around parts of England. Setting off from Trent University in Nottingham, Claire pedalled her way through Leicestershire, Cambridgeshire, Hertfordshire, Oxfordshire, Berkshire and Surrey, finally finishing in London. Along the way, she visited as many schools as possible to tell the children about the impact of her spinal cord injury, how she managed to rebuild her life and about her 17-day marathon. 'I hope to encourage them to believe in themselves and set personal goals to achieve,' she said.

Lomas' trek raised another £85,000, to which she added more than £75,000 in 2014. In October 2015, her fundraising total reached £500,000.

She told the *Daily Mirror* in 2013:

" *So many amazing things have happened to me since I became paralysed that I never dwell on the negatives. I thought my accident would hinder me a lot but it has been the making of me.*

Maickel Melamed – A glorious finish against all the odds

'Raise the bar of your own expectations for yourself. Human power is infinite.'

There are times when last seems better than first. Certainly more of an achievement.

Maickel Melamed (*b*. 1975) is a Venezuelan motivational speaker and teacher, a physiotherapist and a coach. He is also a long-distance runner – and the man who came last in the 2015 Boston Marathon.

Twenty hours after the race started, 39-year-old Melamed, supported by friends and supporters, finally crossed the line at 5 o'clock in the morning – an astonishing achievement for a man barely able to move, let alone walk, because of a rare form of muscular dystrophy.

Even more remarkably, Boston was Melamed's fifth marathon – and his last. His previous marathons had taken too much of a toll on him physically, he explained. He chose Boston as the best place to bow out: the city in which he had received a life-saving operation as a child. Melamed had been given just seven days to live at birth: Boston gave him life; and 39 years later, Melamed celebrated that life with the city – and with the entire running world.

The weather was appalling; even so there were crowds to see Melamed finish. His triumph over his own personal adversity struck a huge chord in a city and at a race that had been rocked by the Boston bombings just two years before.

Speaking at a Boston City Hall reception to mark his achievement, Melamed said:

> *After 20 hours of rain, wind and cold, Boston is still strong. The whole city has been so helpful and loving. The message here is that love is so much stronger than death. It was an honour to run the streets of this city.*

Although Boston's hilly track had become particularly tough around mile 24, Melamed's supporters and physical trainers had found a way to keep him going. He would rest for 10 seconds and then take four to six steps, and then he would collapse into his support team's arms, and yet they – and he – would always find a way to continue. Melamed explained:

> *You have to know why you're doing it, because in the last mile, the marathon will ask you if you have a reason, and if you don't have it, you will quit.*

Melamed had previously completed marathons in Chicago, New York, Berlin and Tokyo. He resolved there would be no more after Boston, but he resolved to finish it in style – and with a message for the world. He left it to his childhood friend Natalie Howard to voice it once he had reached his goal:

> *This is not about Maickel, it's not about Venezuela. It's about the world, and it's about creating a world for peace with the intention of putting humanity first.*

Phil Packer – The London Marathon in 14 days

'It's all about what I can do, not about what I can't do.'

British Army major Phil Packer was told he would never walk again after an attack in Basra in February 2008 in which he sustained catastrophic spinal cord injuries. While on operational duty, he suffered a bruised heart, damage to his ribs and chest and the loss of the motor and sensory use of his legs. Psychological trauma compounded the physical.

Packer's response was to rebuild his life through a series of extreme challenges on a journey that has subsequently inspired millions.

Just a year after his injuries, Packer completed the 2009 London Marathon. On crutches, he finished the course in two painstaking weeks. He said the support had been overwhelming all the way round. Olympic legend Sir Steve Redgrave was there at the finish to present him with his marathon medal. Joining him in The Mall were soldiers he had served with in Iraq, Bosnia, Kosovo and Northern Ireland.

He told the *Daily Telegraph*:

> *I really had to steel myself for those last few hundred metres to the finish. Given the loss of life we had heard of in Afghanistan and the colleagues who had gathered at the finish, it was sombre rather than joyous. All I felt was that I have had closure on an event I said I would complete.*

Packer came to the marathon on the back of a number of sporting challenges, including rowing the English Channel in just over 15 hours and completing a skydive. His aim was to raise £1 million for the services charity Help for Heroes.

> *The greatest realisation I've had doing the marathon is that regardless of what happens to you in life, there are still major goals you can set yourself and major achievements to be made. My injury is not a disability to me any more. It's all about what I can do, not about what I can't do. That feeling is very strong.*

In March 2010, Packer retired from the armed forces and now devotes his energies to the British Inspiration Trust (BRIT) which he founded, aiming to build a Residential Centre of Inspiration for charities and their young people. The charity works to transform the lives of young people, aged 16–25, across the UK who are facing trauma and adversity, particularly relating to self-harm, depression and mental well-being.

In the meantime, the challenges have continued. In 2012, Packer walked 2,012 miles in 331 days through every county in Great Britain and Northern Ireland, the equivalent to around 310 marathons. When walking, Packer uses four times the energy of someone without his spinal cord injuries.

> Physically it's been a slog. It's been tough. I've overcooked it on certain days and weeks and paid the cost. [But] it's been one of the most remarkable years I've ever had.

In 2015, Packer, whose achievements have brought him an MBE and the Helen Rollason Award at the BBC Sports Personality of the Year, turned his attention once again to the marathon. Six years after completing a marathon distance in 14 days, this time he finished it in 14 hours, another major fundraiser for his British Inspirational Trust. It was a remarkable improvement. Packer explained: 'The training programme has been very tough. It has been almost 60 weeks of strength and endurance training following on from five years of physical challenges that have led to slight improvements to my mobility.'

His marathon feat was the equivalent of walking 100 miles in a day.

CHAPTER EIGHT

THE 80s GREATS OF WOMEN'S DISTANCE RUNNING

Grete Waitz – Nine-time New York City champion

*'She's the queen of the
road, but she doesn't
behave like a monarch.'*

If Kathrine Switzer opened the door at the Boston Marathon in 1967, you could say that Grete Waitz ran right through it – she is another influential figure in women's distance running who showed the world precisely what women are capable of. The Norwegian won the World Marathon title in 1983, the New York Marathon nine times, the London Marathon twice and the World Cross-country Championship on five occasions.

Mary Wittenberg, president of the New York Road Runners, organisers of the New York City Marathon, underlines her significance to women's running:

> *She is our sport's towering legend. I believe not only in New York, but around the world, marathoning is what it is today because of Grete. She was the first big time female track runner to step up to the marathon and change the whole sport.*

With bronze medals in two European Championships, and two 3,000 m world records to her name, Waitz nearly abandoned her marathon career in 1978 before it had even begun. But her husband, Jack, who was also her coach, persuaded her to run New York City – even though she had never run more than 13 miles before. Effectively, as she admitted, she ran her debut marathon as a lark, for fun, as it were. Jack told her that a trip to New York would be like a second honeymoon for them.

Clearly doubtful she would complete the course, New York City Marathon founder and race director Fred Lebow agreed to bring her in as a pacemaker. It proved an inspired move. Waitz did indeed set the pace and didn't drop out or back as pacemakers generally do. She won the 1978 New York City Marathon in a new women's world record time of 2 hours 32 minutes 30 seconds.

> *When I crossed the line I was furious with Jack because my whole body hurt. But once the anger had gone and the pain had lessened and the victory*

*soaked in, I realised that it was a milestone in
my career.*

Waitz went on to set the world standard three more times. She
returned to New York nine times in the next ten years. Only
once, because of injury, did she fail to win.

In 1979, Waitz finished the race in 2:27:33, beating her own
record by almost 5 minutes — an achievement which made her
officially the first woman to run a marathon in under two and
a half hours. But 1983 was Waitz's greatest year. She set a new
world record in the London Marathon; won the World Marathon
title in the inaugural championships in Helsinki; and ended the
year with her fifth New York victory. She continued to clock up
the New York victories and added another success in London in
1986 before retiring from serious racing in 1991.

In 1992, she teamed up with her friend Fred Lebow one final time
to run his home course together. Lebow was being treated for brain
cancer, which was then in remission. Their time was 5:32:35. Before
the race, Lebow said: 'I always say she's the queen of the road, but she
doesn't behave like a monarch.' Waitz would always call it her tenth
victory in New York. Lebow succumbed to his cancer in 1994.

In 2005, Waitz was herself diagnosed with cancer. In her last
years, Waitz worked tirelessly for the Norwegian cancer charity
Aktiv Mot Kreft (Active Against Cancer) before her death on
19 April 2011 at the age of 57. She was buried in Norway at the
state's expense as a mark of honour.

The *New York Times*, in the city whose race she made her own,
lamented a runner 'whose humility and athleticism made her a
singularly graceful champion and a role model for young runners,
especially women'. Marathon world record holder Paula Radcliffe
mourned 'an amazing champion and more amazing person'.

Grete Waitz's running achievements

1988, 1986, 1985, 1984, 1983, 1982, 1980, 1979, 1978	New York City Marathon	Winner
1984	Los Angeles Olympics, marathon	Silver
1984	15,000 m	47:53 (WR)
1983, 1981, 1978	World Cross-country Championships	Winner
1983, 1980, 1979, 1978	Marathon world records	2:25:29, 2:25:41, 2:27:33, 2:32:30
1983	World Marathon Championships	Winner
1980	10,000 m	31:00 (WR)
1979	10 miles	53:05 (WR)
1976	3,000 m	8:45.4 (WR)
1975	3,000 m	8:46.6 (WR)

Ingrid Kristiansen – The other half of a great rivalry

'If she can do it,
I can do it too.'

Pose the question 'who is the greatest woman long-distance runner of all time?', and it won't be long before the name Ingrid Kristiansen surfaces.

Kristiansen's background was as an elite Nordic skier, a discipline that arguably gave her the fitness to make the move across to long-distance running. As a cross-country skier, she ran a great deal during the year in preparation for the ski season. The transition to running was straightforward, and the Norwegian-born Kristiansen went on to become the first athlete to win world titles in all three running disciplines: track, road and cross-country.

In a sparkling career, Kristiansen (*b.* 1956) won the London, Boston, New York City and Chicago Marathons and also simultaneously held the world records at 5,000 m (14:37.33), 10,000 m (30:13.74) and the marathon (2:21:06). More than 30 years on, her marathon best would still be highly competitive at marathons around the world.

Kristiansen also won the Stockholm Marathon three times and at Houston twice. As for that single win in New York, some of her supporters still argue that she was never given a fair crack in a city where Grete Waitz was allowed to dominate. In 2013, Kristiansen's husband, Arve, claimed Ingrid was left uninvited to many New York races simply to assure the continued success of her Norwegian rival – a claim swiftly dismissed by NYC Marathon organisers, the New York Road Runners. They issued a statement:

> *Ingrid was invited many times to the New York City Marathon with all of the other great runners of that time. The New York City Marathon has always been an inclusive and welcoming event and we continue to work to expand access to this great race.*

The relationship between Waitz and Kristiansen was certainly an interesting one, as Kristiansen admitted in an interview with *Sports Illustrated* in 1986:

> *She was not my ideal, in the sense that I wanted to imitate everything about her, but she showed what women could do if we trained like men. She showed that Norwegian girls can beat the best. It was frustrating to be behind her for those years, but there was always the feeling, 'If she can do it, I can do it too'.*

Whatever the truth of her husband's New York allegations, Kristiansen's results speak for themselves. At least 11 times she ran under the 2:30:00 benchmark in marathons.

Kristiansen now works in fitness training and in preparing others for the marathon, on the back of her own impressive credentials. History will judge her alongside her rival and contemporary Waitz as a truly major figure in the development and encouragement of women's long-distance running.

Ingrid Kristiansen's personal bests

19 March 1989	New Bedford, MA	Half-Marathon	1:08:31
21 November 1987	Monaco	15,000 m	47:17
13 August 1986	Zürich	3,000 m	8:34.10
5 August 1986	Stockholm	5,000 m	14:37.33
5 July 1986	Oslo	10,000 m	30:13.74
21 April 1985	London	Marathon	2:21:06

Rosa Mota – Olympic dreams

*'It was worth all
that work.'*

Rosa Mota was part of the great 1980s generation of women marathon runners alongside Joan Benoit Samuelson from the United States and the Norwegian rivals Grete Waitz and Ingrid Kristiansen – names which probably come to mind before Mota's does. But when the Association of International Marathons and Distance Races met in 2012 to honour the best woman marathoner of all time, Mota was their choice.

Hers was a stellar career, packed with firsts and boasting an astonishing marathon-to-victory conversion rate. Winner of the first official international championship marathon for women, she ran 21 major marathons between 1982 and 1992 and won no fewer than 14 of them.

Mota's debut was at the 1982 European Championships in Athens where she beat Ingrid Kristiansen to take the title in her very first marathon. Running against the strongest women's marathon field ever assembled two years later, she won bronze in the first women's Olympic marathon in Los Angeles in 1984. It immediately started her thinking about the Seoul Olympics four years later.

> When I won the bronze medal it made me really happy because I didn't expect to make the podium, and it was Portugal's first Olympic medal among the female athletes. I started to think that I had four years to prepare myself for Seoul. I started working the day after the Los Angeles Marathon because you can't prepare for a race in one day. You have to prepare for a race over many years, and I started thinking about Seoul right away.

Having won the Chicago Marathon in 1983, Mota won it again in 1984, just months after the Olympics, lowering the course record by a huge 5 minutes. When she returned to the Chicago Marathon in 1985, she ran a career best of 2:23:29, a time that brought her third place on the day. Mota went on to be crowned European Champion again in 1986 and World Champion in 1987. Her preparation for the Seoul Olympics was looking good, and her preparation paid off. In Seoul, Mota took gold to become the first woman to win multiple Olympic marathon medals. She also became the only woman to be simultaneously the reigning Olympic, World and European champions.

> *Entering the stadium is an unforgettable moment. Here I'm just 400 metres away from being the Olympic champion. When I entered the stadium, I looked back. I was on my own, and I thought I was close to victory. Now it's 300 metres, and I've already started to see the finish line from the other side. I'm entering the home straight, and I'm going to become Olympic champion. It's a moment of joy, of happiness which stays forever in my memory, in my heart. This is something you don't forget. It was worth all that work.*

Mota, who won the Boston Marathon three times in all (1987, 1988 and 1990), retired from marathon running after failing to finish the 1992 London Marathon due to a stomach problem. Still considered an ambassador for her sport, she enjoys enduring popularity in Portugal. In 2004, she carried the Olympic flame along the roads of Athens before the summer Olympics.

Rosa Mota's marathon victories

1991 London Marathon	2:26:14
1990 European Championships Split	2:31:27
1990 Boston Marathon	2:25:24

1990 Osaka Marathon	2:27:47
1988 Olympic Games Seoul	2:25:40
1988 Boston Marathon	2:24:30
1987 World Championships Rome	2:25:17
1987 Boston Marathon	2:25:21
1986 European Championships Stuttgart	2:28:38
1986 Tokyo International Women's Marathon	2:27:15
1984 Chicago Marathon	2:26:01
1983 Chicago Marathon	2:31:12
1983 Rotterdam Marathon	2:32:27
1982 European Championships Athens	2:36:04

Joan Benoit Samuelson – A giant among runners

'I had an innate desire to succeed.'

The inaugural women's Olympic marathon at the Los Angeles games in 1984 needed a worthy winner. It found one in Joan Benoit Samuelson. Known to the world simply as Joanie, she was named by *Competitor Magazine* 'the greatest American female marathoner of all time'.

Born in 1957, Benoit first began running as part of the recovery process from a leg injury she picked up while skiing. She excelled at athletics at college, and in 1977 she accepted a running scholarship to North Carolina State where she went on to earn All-America honours. But it was in the 1979 Boston Marathon, while still a comparative unknown, that she made her mark. Benoit won in 2:35:15, setting an American record on the tough Boston course; four years later, she was back in Boston to knock more than 2 minutes off the world record to finish in 2:22:43. Her run was considered one of the greatest marathon performances of all time.

The Olympic marathon beckoned, but Benoit suffered an immediate setback. She injured her knee while training for the US women's Olympic marathon trials. An operation was inevitable, and the implications were potentially huge. She went into the operation not knowing if she would ever run again. In fact, she was back on the training track within days. And just 17 days after arthroscopic knee surgery, she won the trials race in Olympia, Washington in 2:31:04. With fellow US qualifiers Julie Brown and Julie Isphording, she had earned her place in the Los Angeles Olympics.

Expectation was huge as the starters – 50 women from 28 countries – stood ready at Santa Monica College at 8 a.m. on 5 August 1984. All the greats of the era were there, including the Norwegians Grete Waitz and Ingrid Kristiansen, New Zealand's Lorraine Moller, Great Britain's Priscilla Welch and reigning European champion, Portugal's Rosa Mota. The gun went, and Benoit ran a daring race.

> *All the commentators thought I made an error and a stupid mistake and they didn't think I knew what I was doing [...] The gun went off and we were in a pack and I wasn't running very efficiently. I was taking smaller steps. I was getting tripped up. There was the first water station and I said, 'Forget this. I am going to find my own space and run my own race.' That is what I did.*

Inspired by the sheer strength of the field, Benoit produced one of the defining women's marathon runs of the era – and on the back of the riskiest of strategies. Benoit made her break after just 3 miles, but the gamble paid off. She ran alone for the final 23 miles to take gold in a time of 2:24:52; Waitz took silver in 2:26:18 and Mota bronze in 2:26:57.

> *The hardest part of the marathon was staring Bill Rodgers in the face the whole time because he was on course doing the commentary so he was on a motorcycle in front of me. I wanted to have a conversation, but they would have thought that he was coaching me, and that's illegal. So I couldn't talk. I wanted him to say how far behind me they were.*

The significance of Benoit's run is underlined by the effect it quickly had. Running USA statistics say around 14,300 women completed a marathon in the US in 1980, comprising roughly 10 per cent of finishers. By 2013, 232,600 women ran a marathon, making up around 43 per cent of finishers. There is no doubt Benoit accelerated the trend, just as she inspired much of the new industry that quickly grew up to provide not just women's kit, but women's races to run.

Benoit hadn't been part of the campaign to stage a women's marathon in the Olympics, but her example inspired women to build on the opportunity it brought, and it wasn't long before she was living up to her billing as an Olympic champion. Her 1985 Chicago Marathon victory set a new American record (2:21:21), which stood until 2003. Benoit still holds the fastest times by an American woman at the Chicago Marathon and Olympic Games.

International marathon highlights

Year	Event	Place	Time
1979	Boston Marathon	1	2:35:15
1981	Boston Marathon	3	2:30:17
1983	Boston Marathon	1	2:22:43
1984	Los Angeles Olympic Marathon	1	2:24:52
1985	Chicago Marathon	1	2:21:21
1988	New York City Marathon	3	2:32:40
1991	Boston Marathon	4	2:26:54
1991	New York City Marathon	6	2:33:49

CHAPTER NINE

WHEN THE MIND IS WILLING

Kim Stemple – With strength to share

'I run it for everyone that thinks that they can't, that thinks that a diagnosis is an end, that thinks their life is over.'

In an initiative that has captured the imagination of thousands, American runner Kim Stemple has been sharing her medals among those who need encouragement – a campaign which has gained huge momentum in what Kim knows will be her own final months.

In 2009, Stemple was a cross-country coach, a special education teacher and a keen marathoner and triathlete. But then she fell ill. Initially flu or pneumonia was suspected, but after three years, a rare mitochondrial disease was finally diagnosed, the cause of the progressive mental and physical deterioration she now knows will kill her. Over the next few years Stemple's doctors uncovered more and more problems including lupus, benign bone tumours, lymphoma and a painful nerve condition. Step by step, her body was gradually failing her.

When her condition prevented her from competing in the 2012 Rock 'n' Roll Marathon in Las Vegas, Stemple lapsed into depression – so a friend who ran the race gave Stemple a finisher's medal, a gift which changed Stemple's whole outlook on life. She hung the medal by her hospital bed where it proved a conversation starter and began to pull her back from the brink of despair.

> *All the other patients thought it was so cool, and I'm like if you like this one, I've got a whole box of them at home.*

Stemple thought about her own race medals, reflected that she wouldn't be taking them with her when she died and resolved to offer them as gifts, hoping they would bring others the same joy the Vegas medal had given her. In that moment, We Finish Together was born, an organisation dedicated to connecting runners and their medals with those who might appreciate a gift. Recipients are simply anyone in need, be they cancer sufferers, children with autism, veterans suffering from PTSD or others who just need to know they are not alone. As the website explains, all the medals in the scheme are donated by a community of runners, swimmers and triathletes across the US, each to be given with a handwritten ribbon message and a handmade tag to someone 'who needs to know they have the support and care that they may need to get them through whatever challenges face them'. As Stemple explained:

> **"** It's that you hold the strength of
> that medal, everything that it took
> to get it, be it a racing medal, a
> gymnast medal, a spelling bee medal.

Stemple described the idea as truly organic, in that it has grown completely naturally. There is no money attached to any of it. The only rule is that it has to be done with love and kindness. Inevitably, the movement quickly gathered momentum, particularly when 51-year-old Stemple declared the fortieth annual Marine Corps Marathon in October 2015 would have to be her last. A marine wife, she said the Marine Corps Marathon, through Virginia and DC, meant the world to her, but it was the end of the road for her as far as marathons went. Now on weekly chemotherapy, Stemple finished it in 4 hours 15 minutes, a personal best by 2 minutes.

As she told *Runner's World*:

> **"** I am going to die; we are all going
> to die – I just have a little different
> perspective on it. So, I'm doing what
> makes me happy instead of lying on the couch
> looking at the loose hair on the pillow.

Patrick Finney – The first runner with MS to complete a marathon in every US state

'It's been an amazing
journey, and I'm on
top of the world.'

On New Year's Day 1998, Texas software engineer Patrick Finney woke up with numbness in his legs. Doctors diagnosed multiple sclerosis and told him to take his medicine and 'take it easy'. Having recently taken up running to shed some weight, Finney declined their advice and persisted with a routine of moderate running. However, his condition steadily deteriorated, and by 2004, he was unable to walk.

Seven years later, after one of the most remarkable comebacks in racing history, 48-year-old Patrick finished the Bellingham Bay Marathon in Washington state, completing his fiftieth marathon in his fiftieth different state, the first person with multiple sclerosis to do so.

Between 1999 and 2011 Finney endured numerous relapses, each one leaving him virtually paralysed until he managed to fight his way back to health. Through rehabilitation therapy and new medications, he managed to regain his ability first to stand and then to walk and eventually to run.

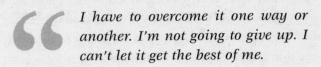

I have to overcome it one way or another. I'm not going to give up. I can't let it get the best of me.

Finney entered a half-marathon in Dallas in 2005 with the sole aim of finishing – and he did so, in just over 4 hours, enough to embolden him to tackle a full marathon the following year, the start of a remarkable run which in January 2010 became a very specific ambition: a marathon in every state before he turned 50.

Finney mapped out marathon dates in every state, compared courses and accelerated his plans to the tune of 40 marathons in 2010. At one point he did 23 marathons in 16 weeks. In the end, at the age of 48, he beat his goal by two years.

And he didn't stop there. The Napa Valley Marathon in March 2013 was Finney's hundredth marathon. Mid-2015 saw him reach 109 when he finished the Bayshore Marathon in Traverse City.

Elizabeth Maiuolo – 'Getting my heart back to perfect shape'

'I have the honour to declare that I am a runner.'

Born and raised in Buenos Aires, Argentina, Elizabeth Maiuolo graduated as a translator and interpreter, before moving to Philadelphia in 2001. Three years later, at the age of 28, she suffered a heart attack. However, she refused to become a heart patient.

Maiuolo objected to the medication she was prescribed, and she refused to contemplate open-heart surgery. Instead, instinctively, she became a runner. With a string of marathons under her belt, her recovery is now total. She knows what has made the difference, and she has even managed to get the medics to see it her way.

As she told *Women's Health* in November 2011:

> My doctor said that I've made a full recovery. He said most people don't ever fully recover and they don't recover as fast as I did. He actually admitted that it was the running that did it. But it took a lot for him to say it out loud.

Maiuolo, who moved to New York City's Upper East Side in 2005, resolved that her life was now about keeping the doctors and the pills away. A regular runner in the New York City Marathon, she left the language industry in 2011 to work full-time in sports training.

She coached for Girls on the Run and worked at Team in Training as a campaign manager before moving on to Autism Speaks as a development manager. Maiuolo has gone on to become a noted blogger at *Runners World Online* and now works as a running gear tester/reviewer and sports social media consultant.

Some might see recklessness in her refusal to follow medical advice. For Maiuolo, it was all about regaining control. She insists that it was running that made her subsequent career possible. As she says on her blog, *RunningAndTheCity*, something like a heart attack seems to snatch control away, leaving you feeling you have little or no grasp on what is happening. Running proved her way back not just to physical health, but also to emotional health. It also opened the door to all the adventures that have followed:

> *Running has taken me into amazing adventures, including the Boulder Bolder (a 10k with 55,000 people at 5,000 feet altitude), the Mountain Madness 50k (where I broke my arm, tore a rotator cuff, broke two ribs, just two weeks before the New York City Marathon!), the Knickerbocker 60k (nine dizzying loops in Central Park!), the Empire State Building Run Up (amazingly lung searing!), the North Face 50k Endurance Challenge at Bear Mountain (wildness and snakes!), and many more races in other cities and countries, with amazing friends and elite runners! Running has not only made me the healthiest I have ever been (plus getting*

my heart back to perfect shape!) but it's made me unmeasurably happy and changed my life completely.

Michael LaForgia – Overcoming double amputation

'I am a better man than I was before.'

Michael LaForgia completed the New York City Marathon in 2002 and 2004 with a personal best of 4 hours 57 minutes. Within weeks, his life changed dramatically for the worse.

IT manager Michael, a 40-year-old father of three, was celebrating the New Year in December 2004 with his family in Maine. He woke in the middle of the night with an excruciating headache, nausea and chills. He cut the family trip short and returned to the family home in New York. The next night, his illness worsened; his wife took him to hospital where his organs started to fail. Doctors feared he wouldn't survive the night. The diagnosis was bacterial meningitis.

After an intensive course of antibiotics and eight days in a coma, LaForgia began to pull through. However, surgeons had to amputate his right leg below the knee and part of his left foot. Two months in hospital and five months in rehabilitation followed, and slowly he was able to make a return to running, this time as a New York advocate for America's National Meningitis Association.

LaForgia's return to running brought a return to the New York City Marathon. Five years after completing the course as an able-bodied runner, he entered in November 2009 as a double amputee, running to raise awareness of the need to promote meningitis prevention. He was a runner on a mission, as he explained to *Runner's World*:

> *It is important to me that I prove to myself and others that I (and other disabled people) can accomplish anything that an able-bodied person can. I want to show that there is no normal, and anyone, regardless of physical capabilities, can achieve greatness. The NYC Marathon was a significant accomplishment for me prior to becoming ill. In completing it with quality I can prove to myself and others that I am a better man than I was before and still capable of great achievements.*

The last few miles were tough. LaForgia later admitted he almost wished he could drop out as he neared Central Park – the point at which his running partner and physical therapist Phil Kreuter checked his prosthetic. His wife, Donna, ran onto the course to join him for the final 3 miles. '[That final stretch] was humbling because I could walk and he couldn't,' she said. However, he struggled on, and crossed the line in 6 hours 21 minutes. He has since run the marathon for a fourth time.

> *As an amputee or someone who has recovered from bacterial meningitis, anytime you can do something you did before your illness, it gives you great satisfaction because it gives you back some form of normalcy. It's an incredible goal to get back something you were able to do before and maybe even do it better.*

LaForgia now uses his experiences to inspire others, speaking to other amputees and encouraging them to get back on course with their lives. His message is that they can achieve anything they had achieved before; they just might have to do it a little differently. And with that difference, for LaForgia, comes perhaps an increased enjoyment in the race – thanks to the support he now receives.

> *I'm also able to inspire others which is just amazing. A number of people tell me they run because they saw me complete a race. That's an incredible feeling.*

Don Wright – The great survivor

'When I was diagnosed, the standard prognosis was three to five years and out, and that was 12 years ago.'

In October 2015, Don Wright completed his ninety-first marathon, the Marine Corps Marathon. There's nothing remarkable about that – except that it was his ninetieth marathon as a cancer survivor. He immediately started preparing for his ninety-first as a cancer patient.

About a year after he took up running to improve his health, and shortly after he ran his first marathon on 21 June 2003, Wright went to the doctor because of back pain. The shocking diagnosis was multiple myeloma, a blood cancer that affects cells in the bone marrow. In the next 12 years, he ran 90 more marathons, all while on active treatment – a number he is determined to add to as he moves towards his target of 100.

Wright has become a hero of the cause for the Patients Rising advocacy group, a body which fights for faster regulatory approvals for new cancer drugs and greater insurance coverage to help terminal patients and their families handle the cost. Patients

Rising see Wright as a living example of what funding and research can achieve. For Wright, it's all about giving a face to the need for more cancer research and for greater access for patients to groundbreaking treatment. Hence linking up with Patients Rising.

In 2008, Wright began taking the experimental drug pomalidomide (now approved and called Pomalyst). For Wright, it was a game changer:

> *My treatment is not your grandfather's chemotherapy. For seven of the last 12 years, I took a pill to manage my cancer. Imagine, a pill to treat cancer! I didn't lose my hair, I didn't lose my lunch and I was able to keep running. That's what research can accomplish.*

Wright's daughter and his wife of more than 50 years travel with him and run half-marathons so they can spend what he calls their golden years together. His progress can be followed on Facebook and Twitter under the banner Race Cancer as he moves towards his century of marathons as a cancer survivor.

Along the way, he has already achieved 50 States Marathon Club membership, finishing at least one marathon in all 50 states. He has insisted all along: running is a key part of keeping healthy.

> *Every single doctor that has treated me encourages me to keep running. A good healthy lifestyle… I think everybody agrees it helps improve the immune system.*

We know running is good exercise, but for Don Wright it has proved to be even more than that. His doctors have now given up predicting how long he might live.

Mark McGirr – Running back from the dead

'Every day is a bonus
day for me. Life is a gift.'

The moral is: if you're going to have a heart attack during a race, make sure there is a doctor in front of you and a nurse just behind you. It was the saving of Oregon's Mark McGirr in the 2014 Rock 'n Roll Oasis Vancouver Half-marathon.

Other than having high cholesterol, 61-year-old McGirr, who runs a family-owned rug and carpet business, had no warning signs that his heart was in danger. A runner off and on for 50 years, he considered himself to be fit and healthy.

His own account of what happened next is shockingly down to earth:

> *Flopped flat on my face like a sack of potatoes. My brain just stopped; my heart stopped. It turned the lights off. I was dead before I hit the ground, is what they say.*

Jack Jay, a doctor at Burnaby Hospital, was running just ahead of McGirr when he collapsed. Sheila Finamore, a nurse at the hospital where Jay worked, was just behind. They stopped and alternated cardiopulmonary resuscitation for 20 to 25 minutes.

Jay later described his experience:

> *I heard this guy go down. I thought he tripped. When we went to help him up, I thought he just twisted*

an ankle. Turns out he was unconscious, in
cardiac arrest. No pulse. No breathing.

McGirr's wife was waiting at the finish line and had no idea that her husband, who was alone in a crowd of thousands, had suffered a heart attack or even that he was at risk of heart disease. A paramedic arrived by bike, and McGirr's pulse and heartbeat were revived with the aid of a defibrillator. McGirr was taken to hospital. As Jay succinctly said: 'He basically came back from the dead.'

Remarkably, even though his heart stopped for 25 minutes, McGirr suffered no brain damage. Within six weeks, he was jogging on a treadmill. McGirr's rehab lasted two months. Before long, he was running 25–30 miles a week – and looking forward to running (and this time completing) the second Rock 'n' Roll Oasis Vancouver Half-marathon.

McGirr had taken to calling the 2015 race his first birthday, and as he stood at the start line with Jay at his side, he wore the same shirt he had worn the year before, stitched up after the medics had ripped it open. McGirr knew his return to the race was against all the odds, but he made it, a key moment in a life he nearly lost.

McGirr had unreserved praise for his saviours:

They're so modest, but they are my
heroes. They're my new best friends
and we're family now.

McGirr's new message to everyone is to learn hands-only CPR. Jay agrees: 'You just push hard and you push fast. If you're not tired after a minute, you're not doing it right.'

CHAPTER TEN

PUSHING THE LIMITS OF HUMAN ENDURANCE

Ted Jackson – Seven in seven on seven for MS

'Ted, we salute you!'

Ted Jackson pulls no punches. He's hard on himself. Fifteen years ago, he says, he was a boozer, a smoker, obese, idle and loathsome: 'Think John Belushi in *Animal House*.'

The turnaround couldn't be more dramatic. He is now a teacher, mentor, fundraiser and extreme event addict. Under his belt, he can boast the Marathon des Sables and also the World Marathon Challenge, seven marathons in seven days on seven continents, completed in the hope of raising £777,000 for the charity Overcoming Multiple Sclerosis. His inspiration is his wife, Sophie, who was diagnosed with the neurological condition in 2009:

> *I was determined to complete the seven marathons for my childhood sweetheart. She means the world to me, our family was left devastated when she was first diagnosed with multiple sclerosis [...] I signed myself up for the event without thinking. I'm not athletic at all. That's why I wanted to do it, to prove that if I can do it anyone can. I put myself in a position where failing wasn't an option. I often sign up to things without thinking but thankfully I'm stubborn and determined enough to power through.*

The World Marathon Challenge offers the supreme logistical and physical challenge. For Jackson, the first marathon began within the Antarctic Circle on 17 January 2015, after which there were just 168 hours left to complete the challenge. During the seven-day time period, competitors had to run marathons at Union Glacier (Antarctica), Punta Arenas (Chile), Miami (USA), Madrid (Spain), Marrakesh (Morocco), Dubai (United Arab Emirates) and Sydney (Australia), thus completing marathons on the planet's seven continents: Antarctica, South America, North America, Europe, Africa, Asia and Australasia. Wide temperature fluctuations, worsening jet lag and extreme fatigue are their enemies.

Sporting the twirling moustache and big, bushy beard of a Victorian adventurer, Jackson, a 42-year-old schoolmaster from Surrey, admitted to nerves as he contemplated going to the ends of the earth for his wife.

As he contemplated the ordeal, Jackson told the *Independent*:

> *I am absolutely terrified, but I am also very excited. [...] I know there will be a moment when I will be in tears, when I think, 'Oh my God, what have I done?' Then I will have to think of Sophie and get through it.*

With Sophie in mind, Jackson duly completed his World Marathon Challenge, taking more than 45 hours to finish the marathons and raising over £160,000 as he did so.

Looking back, he recalled the Antarctic marathon was the most interesting, not least because getting there is so difficult. Once there, you have to deal with the extreme cold. The hardest marathon, however, was day five in Marrakesh, fatigue taking hold after three marathons in the space of 37 hours. A highlight came in the Dubai marathon when he took a break from the road to sing 'Nessun Dorma' for a couple that was getting married on the beach. The reward at the end of it all, at the last of his seven finishing lines, was to be met in Sydney by Professor George Jelinek, from the Overcoming Multiple Sclerosis charity.

Jackson later commented:

> *It is such an awful disease that millions of people suffer from, but the charity changed our lives and that's why I became so adamant to raise so much money for them. [...] There used to be a cloud hanging over her head but the charity has really helped her so I wanted to do as much as I could to raise awareness.*

Angela Tortorice – The women's record for the most marathons in a year

'Running gives me a great sense of freedom and complete control over myself. I live for the runner's high!'

A single marathon is the highlight of the year for hundreds of thousands of marathon runners. For some, it's the highlight of a lifetime. But Angela Tortorice is no ordinary runner. For a whole year from 1 September 2012, Tortorice pushed herself to run an eventual average of 2.4 marathons a week. When she crossed the finish line in Pocatello, Idaho on 31 August 2013, she completed her one hundred and twenty–ninth marathon in three hundred and sixty-five days, a new women's world record. The previous record was 120. Add up the distances, and that's 3,379 miles in marathons in a single year.

I have a girlfriend that just keeps calling me 'Nuts! You're nuts!' So I get a little bit of that!

Angela ran her first marathon in San Antonio in November 1997 after three years of regular running. Afterwards she admits she found herself thinking, 'I'm never going to do this ever again as long as I live. What was I thinking?' But it wasn't long before she was asking herself, 'Okay, what's next?' Her second marathon followed just a month later, in December. Before long, her aim was to run a marathon in all 50 states. She'd clocked up Chicago, New York and a few others when she met a member of the 50 States Marathon Club. He gave her all the encouragement she needed to carry on and complete the set.

By now, Angela's focus was changing. It was no longer about the time goals, but rather the number of marathons. 'It is hard to mix speed and distance when you are running marathons so close together,' she commented, lamenting her principal injury: 'The credit card is hurting. It has an overuse injury. I've definitely gone through a lot of savings.'

It wasn't an injury she decided to treat by holding back. The marathons kept on coming, and before long she was lining up the record for the most marathons by a woman in a year. By April 2013, Angela, an accountant by profession, had completed 106 marathons within 365 days; and a plan was hatched – even though she was still working full-time.

> "I'm persistent. If I make up my mind, I'm not going to give up. I began to wonder if I could break the record. I started adding up the numbers. I realised I could get 121. I knew I wanted a little bit of a cushion.

Along the way, Angela wore out numerous pairs of shoes and continued adding to that credit card bill, but the end result rewarded her every step and every dollar she had spent. At the age of 46, she secured her record. In doing so, she took her own personal tally of marathons to more than 420. Surprisingly, Tortorice calculated there were still 15 to 20 women with more marathons to their name – though not in the 365-day span she had made her own.

Nor probably with the same sense of enjoyment.

As she told *D Magazine* in 2012:

> You think, 'Am I going to make it today? Am I going to finish?' But there's always somebody out there new you can meet, and there are old friends that are out there. You can have a great time entertaining one another. We tell the same old jokes or make up new ones. We're just having a great time.

Dean Karnazes – The man who can run forever

'I run because if I didn't, I'd be sluggish and glum.'

There are runners whose efforts are genuinely mind-boggling; probably none more so than the Californian ultramarathon man Dean Karnazes. At times it seems he can run forever.

Among his accomplishments, he has continuously run 350 miles, foregoing sleep for three nights; he has run across Death Valley in 50°C (122°F) temperatures; he has run a marathon to the South Pole in −40°C (−40°F); and on ten different occasions, he's run a 200-mile relay race solo, racing alongside teams of twelve. *Men's Fitness* was possibly stating the obvious when they hailed him as one of the fittest men on the planet.

As he says in his book, *Ultramarathon Man: Confessions of an All-Night Runner*:

> I run because if I didn't, I'd be sluggish and glum and spend too much time on the couch. I run to breathe the fresh air. I run to explore. I run

to escape the ordinary. I run to savour the trip along the way. Life becomes a little more vibrant, a little more intense. I like that.

Among numerous other feats of extreme endurance, Karnazes (*b.*1962) also ran 50 marathons, in all 50 US states, in 50 consecutive days, finishing with the New York City Marathon which he ran in 3 hours flat. Tests confirmed Karnazes could do it because he had a body that could take it. Over the course of the 50 marathons, his body adapted to his running schedule to the point that running 183 miles a week caused no more muscle damage than everyday walking for the rest of us.

For Karnazes, it is all about feeling alive:

> *People think I'm crazy to put myself through such torture, though I would argue otherwise. Somewhere along the line we seem to have confused comfort with happiness. Dostoyevsky had it right: 'Suffering is the sole origin of consciousness.' Never are my senses more engaged than when the pain sets in. There is a magic in misery. Just ask any runner.*

Making it all possible is the fact that Karnazes has never experienced any form of muscle burn or cramp. He told the *Guardian* in 2013:

> *At a certain level of intensity, I do feel like I can go a long way without tiring. No matter how hard I push, my muscles never seize up. That's kind of a nice thing*

if I plan to run a long way [...] To be honest, what eventually happens is that I get sleepy. I've run through three nights without sleep and the third night of sleepless running was a bit psychotic. I actually experienced bouts of 'sleep running', where I was falling asleep while in motion, and I just willed myself to keep going.

Karnazes puts his abilities to practical use in the community. His foundation, KARNO KIDS 'provides direct financial support to organisations and programmes that are focused on improving the health and wellness of our youth and restoring and preserving the environment and urban open spaces'.

Stefaan Engels – A year in marathons

'I don't regard my marathon year as torture. It is more like a regular job.'

Former graphic designer Stefaan Engels has been dubbed Marathon Man, and fair enough. In February 2011, he completed a marathon year that was exactly that, a marathon a day for 365 days.

The 49-year-old set off from his home town of Ghent in Belgium on 5 February 2010, went through Portugal, Canada, Mexico, Britain and the United States and crossed his finish line in the Carretera de les Aigues race in Barcelona, 15,400 km later.

His best marathon time was 2 hours 56 minutes. His average marathon time was around 4 hours – impressive going for someone who'd been told as a child to avoid sport.

He told *Time Magazine* in 2011:

> *I was born with asthma. The doctors and my parents said, 'Stay home. It's not good to run.' But that was never my lifestyle. Thanks to running, I am breathing better.*

The previous record holder for successive marathons was Akinori Kusuda, of Japan, who ran 52 races in a row at the age of 65 in 2009. Engels stormed past him – and kept on going for another 313 days – another achievement to add to the fact that he already held the record for the most Ironman triathlons in a year, completing 20 in 2007 and 2008.

> *I recover quickly. I don't run fast and my heartbeat is slow, below 100 if I run 10 kilometres, but it is more a mental story. The problem was thinking about running a marathon every day. I just told myself to run that day and did not think about the next day or next week.*

His achievement has been chronicled in the film *Marathonman 365*, the tale of Engels' record-breaking year in the form of a 52-minute documentary. Film-maker Tom Coeman recorded the doubts, the misery, the triumphs, the happiness and the aggravations which Engels encountered along the way. The film also includes interviews with sports doctor Chris Goossens and clinical biologist Griet Nuytinck in an effort to understand how the body and mind of an ordinary man managed to deliver such an extraordinary performance.

Rob Young – The most marathons in a year

*'I say that with a strong mind and good
heart then the body will follow.'*

You'd expect the world record number of marathons in a year to be 365. Not so. Rob Young, also known as MarathonManUK, managed to fit in 370 – a remarkable feat of endurance.

As he recalls, the change happened overnight, thanks to the inspiration of simply watching the 2014 London Marathon.

He told Sky Sports in 2015:

> *It started off as a bet between my partner and I. We were watching the London Marathon last year and I was really inspired by some of the stories. I said to my missus I could do that. She said I couldn't, and it really went from there. I said I could do 10 or 20 marathons and somehow it got to 50 and off I went. I didn't really know what I was getting myself involved in.*

South Londoner Young set out on his first-ever marathon the very next day. He simply set off and did one around Richmond Park, the start of a journey which took him from an unlikely start, being 'just your average 31-year-old living a regular life in London with my small family', to world record holder status. On 13 April 2015, exactly 365 days after completing his first marathon, he completed his three hundred and seventieth. 'It was an extraordinary feeling,' he reflected, 'knowing I'd run further than anyone else in history' in a single calendar year: more than 10,000 miles.

Young's nine-to-five job meant much of his weekday running was from 3 a.m. to 7 a.m. each morning, with the official marathons ticked off at the weekends. But huge family support played its part, as did the inspiration of the causes he was running for, the NSPCC, Great Ormond Street Hospital and Dreams Come True. He was inspired too by memories of his own painful childhood.

Five years in the Royal Signal Corps had helped Young develop his competitive nature and explore an interest in athletics. But it was community spirit, he says, which inspired him when it came to the longer distances. For Young, marathon running isn't so much an individual pursuit as a joint endeavour, an approach that kept him going in the toughest moments.

Young's explanation for his running success chimes closely with Dean Karnazes'. As he told the *Daily Telegraph*:

> *I don't like saying this stuff about myself, but the scientists say it's because I have a very high pain threshold. I'm very mentally strong. That's the difference between me and most people. They have a point where they'll give up, but I don't have that.*

After 267 marathons, including 28 ultramarathons, in 251 days in the UK, Young crossed the Atlantic to compete in Race Across USA, 3,080 miles from Los Angeles to Washington DC.

Racing in a kilt at his children's request, Young typically completes a marathon in three and a half hours. He insists the task is simple. Mentally he splits each marathon into two segments, treating the first as a race and the second as a cool-down period which means he's ready to do another one the next day or even straight away while staying injury free. Which helps explain why he didn't stop with just the 370 marathons. In the summer of 2015, Young broke the record for the longest ever run without sleep – 373.75 miles (88 hours 17 mins).

Kevin Carr – The fastest man around the world

'It was never meant to come down
to this much of a nail-biter.'

It started and ended at the same spot in Devon – a return that saw 34-year-old Kevin Carr become the first runner to circumnavigate the globe solo. His double achievement was to run around the world in record time and also to become the first person to complete the feat unsupported. Making it a triple achievement was the fact that he undertook it all as part of his battle against depression.

Fitness instructor Carr set off from Haytor, a granite tor on the eastern edge of Dartmoor, in July 2013 and completed one to two marathons a day for the next 19 months on a route which included the scorching heat of deserts, sub-zero temperatures and mountains across 16,300 miles in 621 days. Continually running eastwards, Carr ran coast to coast across four continents and one subcontinent as he closed his own personal loop around the world.

Carr has recounted the journey in his book, *The Fastest Man around the World*, a volume which offers his personal account of his odyssey through 26 countries in the equivalent of 622 full marathons. Twice he entered the Arctic regions, running and camping in temperatures as low as -31°C (-24°F), but he also faced searing temperatures of well over 50°C (122°F). In between times, he climbed the Andes, 12,000 feet high, and ran through canyons.

Carr's route took him through Europe, India, Australia, New Zealand, Canada, USA and South America; dangers along the way included snakes, scorpions, wild dogs, wolves and mountain lions. Most frightening of all, however, was coming face to face with bears in Canada. One of the bears stalked him and then attacked. Carr responded with bear bangers to frighten it away. After three misfires, to his huge relief his fourth attempt sent the bear packing.

The dangers make all the more remarkable the fact that he was the first man to complete the gruelling endurance run unsupported. There was no backup team on hand to help with logistics and arrangements. Instead, Carr had to push or pull everything he needed along the way in various carts, at times weighing more than his own body weight when food and water provisions had to be carried as well. He told the *Daily Mail*:

> *I knew the size of the challenge but it was a little bit more of a headache dealing with the logistics and the traffic. It was a bit harder than I had anticipated and took me a bit longer. I didn't have much time to lament on loneliness as I was concentrating on the traffic and where I was going to sleep that night and find a shop. The worst thing I faced was indifference from fashion-savvy people looking at a sweaty dishevelled man pushing a pram down the road.*

As he crossed his own finishing line, Carr managed by a matter of hours to wrest the record for the fastest circumnavigation on foot from Tom Denniss, of Australia. The record was Carr's by less than one day.

Carr's motivation – after suffering with depression in his late teens and early 20s – was to raise money for mental health charity SANE and the British Red Cross. His aim, he said, was to prove that a mind that is sometimes ill 'is not a weak mind'.

Paul Staso – Keeping a promise to the children

'It was a huge mental and physical challenge.'

Running inspires Paul Staso who in turn inspires others, a man on a mission to open up the pleasures and benefits of exercise via an online classroom he now operates.

Ultrarunner, adventurer, speaker, writer and father of four, Staso is a former fifth grade teacher in the States who now uses the Internet as a window into his adventures, getting teams of students from around the world to run/walk with him virtually as he pounds out the miles on the road for real.

For Staso, it's all a continuation of his monumental 3,260-mile solo run across the United States in 2006, from the Pacific Ocean to the Atlantic Ocean, in only 108 days – a journey on which he averaged 30 miles a day on the hot summer pavements, all in fulfilment of a promise he made to 97 children at Russell Elementary School in Missoula, Montana, where his wife, Vicki, was teaching physical education.

Staso told them that if they ran the equivalent of 3,200 miles during the 2005–2006 school year, then he'd do it for real, a commitment which, for Staso, makes it 'my most special and meaningful running achievement': thousands of miles across 15 states simply because he told fourth and fifth grade students that he would do so. Staso had been chatting with his young daughter,

Ashlin, about fitness levels among children. Ashlin wanted to do something to help get the children in her class more active and fit; in response, Ashlin and her father created a virtual run/walk across America curriculum, from the Oregon coast to the Delaware shore.

Staso's actual run took him over the Northern Rocky Mountains, across the Great Plains, through numerous towns and cities, over the steep Appalachian Mountain Range and past the White House through the second hottest summer ever recorded in America. All the while he was pushing BOB, his sole companion, a jogging stroller containing his gear, food and water. BOB stood for Beast of Burden. When fully stocked, it weighed 80 lb.

Staso's life has since become dedicated to encouraging an active, healthy lifestyle in children, promoting goal-setting and teaching children about locations beyond their school grounds in a fun and challenging way.

Staso followed up his 2006 solo epic in 2008 with 620 miles alone across the state of Montana, and, alone again, in 2009 he ran 500 miles through Alaska. In 2010, he then ran 500 miles solo across Germany, and in 2011 506 miles solo across the Mojave Desert. In doing so, he became the first person to run solo from the south rim of the Grand Canyon to Badwater Basin, Death Valley.

> Why do I do it? For personal adventure and the opportunity to encourage kids to be healthy and fit! I grew up running on track and cross-country teams during my middle school and high school years. While attending the University of Montana in the mid-1980s I began to explore my endurance limits... and never looked back.

Cliff Young – The man who gave us the Young Shuffle

'Yes, I can!'

A number of ultramarathon runners have adopted the Young Shuffle as an energy-efficient means of forward propulsion. Some of them might even know just who the Young in question was – a 61-year-old farmer who became an unlikely hero when he won one of the world's toughest races.

Cliff Young made his mark in 1983 at Australia's most gruelling annual ultramarathon, the 875-km (543.7-mile) endurance race from Sydney to Melbourne. The course is considered among the most demanding in the world. It takes five days to complete and is normally attempted only by world-class athletes who train specially for the event. When Young turned up in his overalls and work boots, everyone thought he was a spectator, but no, he was a competitor, he insisted, ready and willing to take on the challenge. Most competitors were less than 30; Young was double their age. Most competitors turned up with big-name sports-company backing; Young had nothing more than his race number. Could he do it, the press asked. Yes, he could.

> *Yes, I can. See, I grew up on a farm where we couldn't afford horses or tractors, and the whole time I was growing up, whenever the storms would roll in, I'd have to go out and round up the sheep. We had 2,000 sheep on 2,000 acres. Sometimes I would have to run those sheep for two or three days. It took a long time, but I'd always catch them. I believe I can run this race.*

What transpired was a modern-day tortoise and the hare. The other runners quickly left Young behind, but while the others rested, Young ran through the night. Every night while the others slept, Young closed the gap. And then he opened up a gap of his own. The first competitor to cross the line, Young came out of nowhere to defeat the world's best long-distance runners. Young finished the 875-km race in 5 days, 15 hours 4 minutes, setting a new record as he did so.

At the start, one of the media commentators had dubbed him the nation's worst-dressed sportsman; by the end, another was quipping that if they hadn't stopped him, he would simply have kept on going to Perth.

Looking back, Young said simply that when he was running, he imagined he was chasing sheep and trying to outrun a storm. It was the perfect way to keep on going. He quite literally took it all in his stride. When he was handed his prize money, he said he didn't even know there was a prize. He took it but purely so he could give it away to other runners.

Every nation likes a folk hero, and Young was precisely that. In his galoshes, with his shuffling run and his refusal to stop even for sleep, he was a ready-made legend and ran straight into the nation's hearts as huge interest grew up around him. Young left the world-class athletes behind – and all they could do was follow his lead. These days it is standard practice at the race to run through the night if you are serious about winning.

As for his style, which appeared both leisurely and amateurish, more shuffle than run, the general consensus was that there was something distinctly ergonomic about his gait. The Young Shuffle lives on. At least three subsequent champions in the Sydney–Melbourne ultramarathon have used his shuffle to win the race.

Young was at it again in 1997, this time attempting to run all the way around Australia. By now he was 76 years old, but it wasn't his fault he didn't succeed. Young had to call a halt when a crew member fell ill, by which time he had completed more than 6,000 km of the 16,000-km journey.

Young stopped racing at the age of 78 after a mild stroke. He died in 2003 at the age of 81. On his passing, Australian Ultra Runners Association president Ian Cornelius described him as 'an ordinary guy who achieved extraordinary things'.

Marathon Maniac Larry – Record after record

'All runners are optimists.
Pessimists don't run marathons.'

'1,500 marathons and counting…' Four simple words on Larry Macon's Facebook page – four simple words which record one of marathon running's most astonishing achievements.

After breaking four Guinness World Records for the most marathons run in one year, San Antonio lawyer Macon went past the 1,500 mark in 2015, an aggregated distance of 39,300 miles in marathons alone, enough to take him one and a half times around the circumference of the earth.

> *The hard part is travelling from place to place, making connections and going two to three days without sleep. Once you get to the race, you can always run, walk or crawl to finish the 26.2 miles.*

The irony is that it all started with a fib. As Macon recalled in an interview with ESPN, he was chatting with fellow lawyers one day in 1996 about what they had been up to at the weekend. Everyone else had been doing impressive things. Macon didn't like to be the odd one out.

> They said, 'Larry, what did you do?' Well the truth is Larry didn't do anything. He worked all weekend. But I glanced at a newspaper and said, 'Oh, I'm training for a marathon.' Absolute lie. And they said, 'That's three weeks from now. Great, Larry, we'll have a party for you after.' Damn. Caught.

And so he felt compelled to run a marathon. By choice he ran another. And another. And it wasn't long before he ran marathons on successive weekends.

Then came the assault on the record books. Macon ran 105 marathons in 2008, which was recognised as the most ever in a year by Guinness World Records. In 2010, he ran 113 marathons for a new record; in 2012, he smashed past his own benchmark to clock up a grand total of 157.

And then, at the age of 69, capping it all, Larry recorded 255 marathons, at one point running a marathon on 64 consecutive days. Running generally in the 5- to 7-hour range, Macon began his attempt on 1 December 2012 at the Baton Rouge Marathon in Louisiana and completed the last of his marathons at the Dozen Sweet Potatoes PM Marathon in San Antonio, Texas, on 30 November 2013. Along the way, 24 pairs of running shoes bit the dust.

Inevitably, celebrity status has come hot on Macon's heels. News teams caught up with him for his seventieth birthday. They asked him why he would want to spend a landmark birthday out there running in the bitter cold. Not surprisingly, Macon had a ready answer:

> *It's magnificent. It's because we can, because you can challenge yourself. You can have a wonderful day and there's nothing better than running.*

Four years earlier, his hometown website *My San Antonio* tried to nail just what it was that kept Macon running. They described him as being a 'tad on the obsessive side', but with a 'friendly demeanour and a million-dollar smile', maybe the result, they speculated, of a constant firing of endorphins, the addiction of a man who happened to find himself in a Forrest Gump kind of loop: the more he ran the more he wanted to run. Again, the question was why; Macon gave the perfect answer:

> *Because it's so much fun. If you aren't focused on time, you can talk to people all through the race. I've had great conversations with people from all over the world.*

In April 2013, Macon was caught up in the tragedy of the Boston Marathon bombing. He was forced off the course a mile or so from the finishing line. He made his way to a nearby synagogue. After discovering his hotel was off limits, he tried to head to the airport, but his driver couldn't get to him as the way was blocked. Macon recalled, 'I told them, "I've still got another

mile in me, so pick a spot within a mile and I'll run to you.'"
And so, as best he could, he completed his one thousand
and twenty-fifth marathon and his tenth in Boston.

Istvan Sipos – Running to infinity

*'Running is an outer expression of each human
being's personal struggle to achieve perfection.'*

Hungarian ultrarunner Istvan Sipos dreamt of running to infinity.
He fulfilled his dream when he took part in – and won – the
monumental MoonBat TransAmerica Footrace in 1994.

The race covered 2,926 miles in 517 hours over 64 days, passing
through 14 states before finally finishing at the Columbus Circle
entrance to New York's Central Park. Faith kept him going, as did
his dream of experiencing eternity first-hand.

He told the *New York Times*:

> *When I was in Kansas, on Route 36,
> I finally had that experience. It gave
> me so much joy to see only the road
> with all that open space. It was a lot like life:
> eternal space on an eternal road.*

Twelve runners started. Sipos and four others, Dante Ciolfi,
Michiyoshi Keiho, Motohiko Sato and Kawika Spaulding,
completed the trek from Los Angeles to New York. For Sipos, it was
a run that simply couldn't be conceived or comprehended within
the realms of the rational. There had to be that extra dimension.

> *It is not possible to approach this race with a logical mind because it is impossible to comprehend. It is for a spiritual reason. It is like preparing your body for a war.*

But it seems for Sipos he hadn't gone quite far enough. Between 14 February and 3 November 2000, Sipos ran 12,554 miles in his native Hungary at an average of 47.5 miles per day for 264 days.

In the meantime, he was also making his mark in the ultradistance races in New York founded by Sri Chinmoy, an author, musician, artist, athlete and master of meditation. For Sri Chinmoy, the ultimate goal, in running as in everything, was to increase and to enhance our spirituality:

> *My ultimate goal is for the power of love*
> *To replace the love of power*
> *Within each individual.*
> *My ultimate goal is for the whole world*
> *To walk together in peace and oneness.*

And to this end, Sri Chinmoy's students set up the Sri Chinmoy Marathon Team in 1977. The team then set up the race. In 1993, Sipos set a new record in an early 1,300-mile incarnation.

In 1996, the Sri Chinmoy Marathon Team increased the challenge to a 2,700-mile race. Five runners finished the distance within the 47-day time limit. In 1997, the distance was increased again, this time to 3,100 miles to reflect the fact that Sri Chinmoy was born in India in 1931. Two runners finished. In 1998, Sipos was there to join the challenge, the first of four finishers across the line in 46 days 17 hours at a remarkable 66.3 miles per day.

Making the achievement all the more remarkable is the nature of the course itself. Billed as the grand test of endurance and survival, the race demands almost superhuman stamina and concentration from its runners. It also demands an ability to withstand tiredness beyond most mortals. But just as importantly, the competitors need to be able to combat the sheer boredom of going round and round and round – for this is a race like no other. It challenges a small group of athletes to negotiate 5,649 laps of an 883-m course in 51 days. Roughly 115 times a day, the runners run round the Thomas A. Edison Vocational/Technical School in the Queens borough of New York – a site selected because of its broad pavements and closeness to Sri Chinmoy's residence. Certified as the longest footrace in the world, it requires its runners to average 60.7 miles per day if they are to finish within the time limit. Thirty-eight year old Sipos smashed it in 1998.

Sipos was back again in 2008, one of five to finish – much to the amused bafflement of the *New York Times* which called it 'the world's longest sanctioned race, and possibly the most incomprehensible road race ever'. The *Washington Post* also tried to convey the sheer strangeness of it all as the runners ran round and round:

> *From before dawn until well after dark, for 48 days, they have jogged this same, wearying route over asphalt sidewalks, alongside the iron gate that surrounds the school, down a noisy roadway that spits car exhaust and past a dusty baseball diamond. They have run past kids in baggy jeans, idling cars with rap music blaring, and an abandoned black Mazda with no tires, busted windows and everything – from seats to the gas cap – stripped.*

Sipos was once again the winner, crossing the 3,100-mile threshold on the forty-seventh day. His rewards were a trophy and a photo album. The race offers no prize money. Sipos gave himself 5 minutes to savour his victory and then carried on. He didn't even sit down. With a commendable neatness, he wanted to round off his total distance to 5,000 km (approximately 3,106 miles). Another 13 laps remained.

Spreading the word

The UK Sri Chinmoy Marathon Team has been promoting sporting events in the UK since the late 1970s. Events include a 24-hour race in Tooting Bec, London, a 100-km race in Edinburgh, a beginners' triathlon, 2-mile and 10k races and cycling time trials.

The movement is also popular in Australia. In March 2016, there were Sri Chinmoy events in Melbourne, Sydney, Brisbane, Canberra and Jindabyne.

Worldwide, April 2016 events included Bristol, UK; Auckland, New Zealand; Zlín and Prague in the Czech Republic; and Darkhan in Mongolia.

JC Santa Teresa – The most successive ultramarathons

*'I want to do what I can
to bring an end to this
devastating disease.'*

The most consecutive days running an ultramarathon is 21, achieved by JC Santa Teresa, who ran races throughout California and Texas from 10–31 December 2014 – inspired every step of the way by his mother, Delta, a breast cancer survivor.

Santa Teresa, of Rockland County, New York, was raising money for a breast cancer charity, the Susan G. Komen Foundation, by running for 21 consecutive days at a rate of 50 km (31 miles) per day, to make a staggering total of 1,050 km (652.5 miles).

A kick-boxer in his youth, Santa Teresa, originally from the Philippines, gave up the sport when he began working in the environmental health and safety department of the New York City electricity provider Con Edison. To regain lost fitness, he decided to take up running. A key moment in his life came when he put together a bucket list in his 30s, vowing to live his life to the fullest. One of the challenges he listed was running a marathon. He ticked it off in 2000, and the marathons started to flow. In 2012, he decided to run 30 marathons during the year, raising money for breast cancer awareness following his mother's diagnosis a couple of years before.

He was very close to both his parents and felt sure both they and he would live for ever. But in 1999, his father died of emphysema at the age of 61. Eight years later, his mother received her breast cancer diagnosis. For Santa Teresa, the instinctive response was to run – and he prides himself on encouraging others to do the same, with the aim of bringing an end to the disease.

I never thought I'd be running this much. When I started, it was just to try to get in shape.

His mother's illness was also his inspiration for his assault on the ultramarathons, for which he prepared meticulously. Santa Teresa warmed up with an 50-mile run including sections of the Appalachian Trail, just to make it more difficult. Two weeks later, he completed a marathon in Delaware which also included large sections of trail running. Three weeks later, he embarked on his challenge, starting off in Long Beach, California for the first of 13 ultras. He then went to San Antonio, Texas, where he did eight more to run up his 21 consecutive days.

By 2015, at the age of 52, Santa Teresa had completed races in all 50 states and on every continent, averaging more than one marathon per week over a two-year period. His 2015 marathons included Antarctica and Rome; and the marathons just kept on coming.

Santa Teresa explained:

> I'm slowing down, but not physically. I just want to have fun and be social, and, most importantly, be healthy.'

CHAPTER ELEVEN
IN THE TOUGHEST PLACES

Mauro Prosperi – Drinking bats' blood to survive

'Death didn't want me yet.'

It's hard to imagine what drives people to take on the infamous Marathon des Sables. Contestants find themselves in the Sahara Desert with nothing but rolling sand dunes for miles around. As they plough through the sand, a fine dust kicks up, and the runners' lungs feel parched as they struggle through temperatures in excess of 50°C (122°F).

In such conditions, each step becomes a furious mental battle: one part of the brain is screaming out for the runners to stop; the other part for them to soldier on towards the eventual finish – a finish that will come only after the equivalent of nearly six marathons in five or six days and a total distance of some 156 miles.

The Marathon des Sables combines nature at its most savage with challenge at its most extreme: a race so difficult the organisers ask you to specify where you want your body to be sent in the event of your death.

Mauro Prosperi very nearly became its victim when a sandstorm left him lost in the desert for ten days in 1994.

Prosperi was a 39-year-old former Olympic pentathlete who worked for the mounted police in Sicily – and a man hooked on extreme marathons. For Prosperi, the attraction was the closeness they brought him to nature. As a professional athlete, he made the medals his priority; as an extreme runner, he allowed himself to enjoy the mountains, the deserts and the glaciers. The Marathon des Sables seemed perfect as his next challenge.

The race has grown significantly in numbers in the years since it began. In 2015, there were 1,237 finishers. Back in 1994, there were only 80 starters. Getting lost was a real danger, and on the fourth day, things began to go seriously wrong for Prosperi alone in an area of sand dunes.

He told the BBC:

> *Suddenly a very violent sandstorm began. The wind kicked in with a terrifying fury. I was swallowed by a yellow wall of sand. I was blinded. I couldn't breathe. The sand whipped my face. It was like a storm of needles. I understood for the first time how powerful a sandstorm could be.*

It lasted 8 hours. Prosperi settled down to sleep on the dunes. When he woke up, it was to a transformed landscape. He ran for four hours and then realised there wasn't any point running at all. He was lost.

Prosperi knew to save his urine at a point when he was still well-hydrated – potentially life-saving fluid for later. And he knew to walk only in the morning and in the evening when temperatures were at their most tolerable. At one point he sheltered for a few days in a Muslim shrine, known as a marabout, where he had to kill bats and drink their blood to survive.

He was clinging to hope, but when an aeroplane passed by without seeing him, Prosperi began to give in to despair. He knew his body needed to be found for his pension to be paid. He reasoned his best hope of that happening was to die in the shrine – and to accelerate his death.

> *I wasn't afraid of dying, and my decision to take my own life came out of logical reasoning rather than despair. I wrote a note to my wife with a piece of charcoal and then cut my wrists. I lay down and waited to die, but my blood had thickened and wouldn't drain. The following morning, I woke up. I hadn't managed to kill myself. Death didn't want me yet.*

Prosperi took it as a sign. With renewed hope, he walked on, living off snakes and lizards, eating them raw. The survival instinct was reasserting itself, and he was starting to think of himself as a man of the desert. And then it happened. First he saw goats in the distance, and then he saw a young shepherd girl, who ran towards a large Berber tent to warn the women he was coming. They took him in, took care of him and sent for the police. Prosperi was saved, 181 miles off course, 35 lb lighter. Italy gave him a hero's welcome when he finally made it home.

Four years later, Prosperi was back and this time he conquered the Marathon des Sables. In the years since, he has continued to clock up desert marathons.

The Marathon des Sables was conceived in 1984 by French concert promoter Patrick Bauer when he decided to set out for an epic walk in one of the harshest environments on the planet. It was first run in 1986.

Each year the race now attracts more than 1,000 runners, 200 members of the press and a support management team of more than 400.

Moroccan runner Lahcen Ahansal has won ten titles. His brother Mohamad Ahansal has won five titles.

Dave Heeley – Running blind through the desert

'For me, life is about not what you can't do, but what you can do!'

In April 2015, British marathon runner Dave Heeley became the first blind athlete to complete the 156-mile Marathon des Sables, a course across the Sahara Desert known as the 'toughest footrace on earth'.

The super-fit 57-year-old father of three, known to his friends as 'Blind Dave', completed the six-day challenge, running with his provisions on his back through sand dunes, rocks and dried rivers. Contending with temperatures rising to 50°C (122°F) during the day and below freezing at night, the competitors run the equivalent of six regular marathons.

Heeley, from West Bromwich, was running to raise funds for the Albion Foundation, which works with his beloved West Brom football club to use sport to help the local community. Helping him along the way were two guides and friends, Rosemary Rhodes and Tony Ellis. It was a monumental challenge. Heeley rose to it and would go on to encourage others to do the same.

In an interview with British Blind Sport, Heeley said:

> If I had to give advice to other visually impaired people thinking of taking up athletics, I'd say, 'Do it!' It will change your life, build your confidence and give you independence as well as a social life and better well-being. It makes you a bigger part of the community and you never know what else it will bring. It's unbelievable where it might take you!

The Marathon des Sables wasn't Heeley's first dip into the record books. In 2008, he became the first blind man to run seven marathons on seven continents in seven days, the so-called Seven Magnificent Marathons challenge. His route took him from Port Stanley, Falkland Islands (Antarctica), to Santiago, Chile (South America), Los Angeles, USA (North America), Sydney, Australia (Australasia), Dubai, United Arab Emirates (Asia) and Nairobi, Kenya (Africa) before finishing with the London Marathon.

In 2011, Heeley ran ten marathons in ten days, travelling from John O'Groats to Land's End and cycling between each stage. As he recalls, Heeley was always known as the clumsy kid at school and at home. The reason became clear at around the age of ten when he was diagnosed with the eye condition retinitis pigmentosa: he was going blind. It left him with two routes to take, he says on his website: the negative or the positive. He opted for the latter.

'Blind Dave' now works as an inspirational speaker, and is often invited to share his wisdom with charities, football clubs, educational establishments, theatres and businesses. As he told the *Birmingham Mail*:

> For me, life is about not what you can't do, but what you can do! If an old codger like me can make people stop and think, 'If he can do that, then what can we do?', then it makes it all worthwhile.

Engle, Zahab and Lin – 4,000 miles across the Sahara

'And now the expedition has concluded. Successful. Life-changing. Incredible, but true.'

They contended with temperatures rising to more than 50°C (122°F) during the day and dropping below zero at night; fierce winds compounded the searing heat; and inevitably injury and illness played their part, tendinitis, severe diarrhoea and knee injuries all dragging them down.

And yet they managed it.

Often without a paved road in sight. American Charlie Engle, 44, Canadian Ray Zahab, 38, and Kevin Lin, 30, of Taiwan, clocked up the equivalent of two marathons a day over 111 days until they finally secured their place in the history books as the first modern runners to cross the gruelling 4,000 miles of the Sahara Desert.

Getting up at 4 a.m., they would run until lunch, break and then run until 9.30 p.m. And then they would do it again. Again and again and again – a feat which many had insisted was impossible or, at the very least, unwise. Their journey took them across the world's largest desert as they passed through six countries: Senegal, Mauritania, Mali, Niger, Libya and Egypt. Their route also included a 560-mile detour simply to avoid contracting malaria and dysentery.

Helping them on their way was one of the aims of the mission, to raise awareness for the clean water non-profit group H_2O Africa. At several points along the way, the runners stopped near sparsely populated wells to talk with villagers about the difficulties they face finding water. On their journey, they were followed by a film crew chronicling the journey for actor Matt Damon's production company, LivePlanet. Damon, founder of H_2O Africa Foundation, narrates the finished product, the documentary film *Running the Sahara*, using their story as a way to highlight the water crisis in Africa.

Key to the runners' success was learning to adapt to their conditions and in particular to recognise the futility of fighting against the elements served up by the Sahara. A crucial lesson was that the immeasurable power of the continent would always win in the end. Instead, they learned how to work with their surroundings as best they could so as to make the steady progress that each of the 111 days required of their minds and bodies. As they later said, the expedition was characterised by highs and lows, by camaraderie and solitude and by encounters with both the natural wonders and teeming societies of Africa.

The three ran the final stretch on just 4 hours' sleep, past the Giza pyramids and Cairo to the mouth of the Suez Canal. Reaching the Red Sea, they signalled the end of their road by symbolically putting their hands into the water – a cooling moment at the end of the most demanding of odysseys, one which would take a while to process. As Engle said to the *Washington Post*:

> It will take time to sink in... but this is an absolutely once-in-a-lifetime thing. They say ignorance is bliss, and now that I know how hard this is, I would never consider crossing the Sahara on foot again.

Scott Jurek – A modern Pheidippides

'The top ultrarunner in the country, maybe in the world, arguably of all time.'
NEW YORK TIMES

In 2010, Scott Jurek set a new US all-surface record in 24 hours with 165.7 miles, the equivalent of nearly six and a half marathons in one day – for which he was named *USA Today*'s Athlete of the Week. One might feel they were perhaps underplaying it.

Jurek's resume is astonishing. He is the man with victories in nearly all of ultrarunning's elite trail and road events, from the historic 152-mile Spartathlon to the Hardrock 100, from the Badwater 135-mile Ultramarathon to the Miwok 100k. *Ultrarunning Magazine* named him Ultrarunner of the Year three times – worthy recognition for a man who won the Western States 100 Mile Endurance Run a record seven times on the trot from 1999 to 2005.

Sportsmanship and veganism are key to understanding Jurek. He regards himself as a true student and ambassador of his sport, a competitor who will stop and cheer until the last runner comes home. Just as importantly, he does it all on a 100 per cent plant-based diet, the basis, he says, for his superior endurance, recovery and overall health. He has passed on his lessons and experiences in the bestseller *Eat & Run*.

Jurek draws his inspiration from Native American traditions, the running warriors of ancient Greece and the samurai code of Bushido. Clearly it works. He set a course record in the Badwater Ultramarathon, 135 miles through the 50°C (122°F) heat of Death Valley on his first attempt in 2005. He defended his title in 2006 and then embarked on his first of three wins in the Spartathlon in Greece, which commemorates Pheidippides' run from Athens to Sparta.

For the competitors in the Spartathlon, the sheer difficulty of the course is the point of it all. The athletes have to complete 152 miles within the 36-hour time limit.

Billing itself as 'the world's most gruelling race', the Spartathlon runs over rough tracks and muddy paths, crosses vineyards and olive groves, and climbs steep hillsides. The most challenging section of all, however, takes the runners on the 1,200-m ascent and descent of Mount Parthenio in the dead of night. This is the mountain, covered with rocks and bushes, on which it is said Pheidippides met the god Pan. Strong winds and a lack of pathway add to the hazards. Flashing lights mark the way.

The race website describes the difficulties that follow:

> *Over the mountain the last sections are no less energy sapping and exhausting for the runners as they follow a road that winds up and down hills before descending into Sparta. Even the finest*

athletes start hallucinating as they cover these final stages. Having lost all sense of time and reality, they are on automatic as they push their weary bodies on towards the finishing line at the statue of Leonidas. At most, only about a third of the runners who leave Athens end the course in Sparta.

Jurek was the first North American winner of the Spartathlon and still holds the fastest time on the course behind Yiannis Kouros, a Melbourne-based Greek ultramarathon runner who has run the event's four best ever times.

As Jurek told *Impact Magazine*, it's all about knowing how to overcome the inevitable troughs along the (very long) way:

> *Every race has a low point. It's really hard to run 100 miles or 135 miles and not experience the standard bad experience, but the beauty of it is that you have the opportunity to climb out of the low point and remember how you overcame. I've had really low points in Badwater, for instance: I was vomiting, puking my guts out, really having a very difficult time at around 75 miles ... and I revived myself, and I think that's the key.*

Inevitably, huge mental strength is a major weapon in the ultra long-distance runner's armoury. He also needs a few mental tricks. Jurek boasts a number of different approaches. As he told the *No Meat Athlete* website:

"It's like focusing on the task at hand was really key, and not thinking about 'Okay, I'm at mile 50; I have 100 miles to go'. If I were to think about that too much, it really messes with the mind; it can really be devastating. So for me, it was all about little goals.

Jurek's achievements

US record for 24-hour distance on all surfaces (165.7 miles)
Won the Spartathlon three consecutive years (2006–2008)
Won the Hardrock Hundred-Mile Endurance Run with a new record in 2007
Won the Western States Endurance Run seven consecutive times (1999–2005)
Won the Badwater Ultramarathon twice (2005, 2006)
Won the Miwok 100k Trail Race three times (2002–2004), came second three times (2001, 2005, 2006)
Won the Leona Divide 50 Mile Run four times (2000, 2001, 2002, 2004)
Won the Diez Vista 50k Trail Run twice (2000, 2003)
Won the Montrail Ultra Cup series twice (2000, 2003)

Pat Farmer – 'A burning desire to get back to basics'

*'There's a commonality
between human beings
all over the planet.'*

Australian ultrarunner Pat Farmer declares himself 'dedicated to helping humanity'; his feats, however, seem to go beyond the mere human. Farmer served eight years as an Australian Member of Parliament, with three years as Parliamentary Secretary for Education, Science and Training. But it is with his endurance running that he has made his mark globally.

A multiple world record holder, Farmer has run across Australia, New Zealand, Vietnam, the Middle East and North America, raising millions of dollars along the way for causes, including Lifeline, Cancer Council, the Australian Red Cross and Diabetes Australia.

Farmer first started to get noticed as a runner when he secured second place in his first attempt at the Trans America Road Race in 1993; two years later, he was fourth despite running 50 days with a stress fracture in his leg. Four years after that, in 1999, he established the fastest Around Australia Long Run Record of continuous running, completing 14,662.4 km (9,110 mile) during his Centenary of Federation run, lasting 191 days 10 minutes.

In 2011, he topped even that when he made his trek from the North Pole to the South Pole.

On the way, Farmer ran through 14 countries. His efforts raised $100 million for the International Red Cross. His website dedicated to the event, *Pole to Pole Run*, labels it the 'greatest run in history'. Few would argue.

Farmer divided the trek into five sections, successively Arctic, Canada to Panama, Darien Jungle, South America and Antarctica, respectively ice trek, road run, jungle trek, road run and ice trek. The first section took him from the North Pole to Ward Hunt Island, Canada; the second from the most northern road in Quebec to Montreal and Ottawa and then down the USA's east coast into Central America. Section three was from Southern Panama to Northern Colombia; section four from Northern Colombia to Tierra Del Fuego; and the final section, in Antarctica, from Ronne Ice Shelf to the South Pole, a total of 20,919 km (13,000 miles) in ten months, averaging about 46 marathons a month.

And yes, people did doubt his sanity.

> *It's gone beyond the crazy stage. It's this burning desire to get back to basics. To move away from the computer and out of the office; to experience life and walk the path that no one has walked before. Guys will go through a mid-life crisis. They used to buy [a] red Porsche but now it's different. They're looking for more from life. So people get into these adventures – they want to climb mountains, or hike in exotic locations or go trekking through jungles or forests or run in ultramarathons.*

And that probably explains why he still wasn't finished. In 2012–2013, Farmer completed his Pole-to-Pole Vietnam challenge. Once again raising funds for the International Red Cross, this time he ran the length of Vietnam. His 3,000-km (1,860-mile) run, completed with Vietnamese runner Huy Mai, also commemorated the fortieth anniversary of the relations agreement between Australia and Vietnam which cemented bilateral cooperation. Completing the run, he declared himself to be 'looking forward more than anything to an ice cream and a chocolate milkshake'. He reflected:

> *Never has the face of humanity been shown in such a positive light than through this event which has touched the lives not only of the onlookers who have covered the length of Vietnam but also the participants, myself and my crew, who have been moved by the generosity, the physical support and the spirit of the people.*

In 2014, Farmer was off again, embarking on his Middle East Peace Run, 1,500 km (870 miles) to highlight all the problems faced by one of the world's most troubled regions and also to encourage the world to see the region in a new light.

> *I want to show the humanity of those places. If I can do that by simply running and getting people to run with me, I hope they will realise their differences aren't so big. This is an opportunity to get people to turn their words and feelings of peace into action. Sport has a greater opportunity to do that.*

Pat Farmer's other achievements

Twice world record holder for crossing Australia's Simpson Desert
Ranked third in the world for 1,600 km on a track
Ran 2,500 km around New South Wales for charity in 42 consecutive days

Scott and Rhys Jenkins – The hottest place on earth

'The most demanding and extreme running race offered anywhere on the planet.'

Two Welsh brothers managed to break records as they completed a dangerously difficult race through extreme heat. Scott, 34, and Rhys Jenkins, 27, from Penarth, became the first siblings to complete the Death Valley single, with Rhys also becoming the fastest British man to complete the double.

Billed as 'the world's toughest footrace', the Nutrimatix Badwater 135 – the 'single' – covers 135 miles non-stop from Death Valley to Mount Whitney, annually pitting up to a hundred of the world's toughest athletes against one another and against the elements. Its website describes it as 'the most demanding and extreme running race offered anywhere on the planet'. You are running through the hottest place on earth.

The start line is at Badwater, Death Valley, the lowest elevation in North America at 280 feet below sea level. The race finishes at

Whitney Portal at 8,300 feet. Along the way, the course covers three mountain ranges for a total cumulative vertical ascent of 14,600 feet and 6,100 feet of cumulative descent. If you want to do the 'double', you then turn round and go back to the start... which is precisely what the brothers attempted: 270 miles, the equivalent of more than ten back-to-back marathons on just 7 hours' sleep.

Even in normal conditions, it's a feat that seems unimaginable to most of us, but the brothers were running through temperatures above 38°C (100°F), even at night, when they set off on Tuesday 14 July 2015. Death Valley has the hottest recorded air temperature on earth, hovering at around 48°C (118°F) degrees and peaking at 58°C (136°F). Runners run on tarmac reaching temperatures of 93°C (119°F), and if the heat isn't enough, they also have to contend with scorpions, tarantulas, bobcats and kit foxes.

Scott was dogged by injury and could not complete the full distance. Rhys, however, survived to cross the line. He later said that the final 30 miles into a stiff headwind were horrific, but the key was simply to break each part down into small achievable goals, dig deep and keep on moving one foot at a time, fuelled along the way by Pringles, pizza, burgers and extreme sports hydration tablets.

Rhys' aim had been to finish in 96 hours, which would have set a Guinness World Record for the fastest double crossing on foot. In fact, he finished in 107 hours – more than enough to leave brother Scott awestruck.

For the brothers, the achievement was a double one: the first siblings to run Death Valley and the first Welsh people to run Death Valley. A key part of their motivation was to raise money for Save the Children and for Operation Smile which repairs cleft lips, cleft palates and other facial deformities.

The Death Valley run wasn't the brothers' first great adventure. In April 2012, the brothers were among a group of Penarth runners who completed an epic, non-stop, 750-mile run around the entire border of Wales. The Around Wales – Around the Clock – Run team averaged 170 miles a day, with each runner taking turns to cover part of the distance over the four days before finishing back at their starting point, the Norwegian Church in Cardiff Bay. Rhys and his brother Scott have also completed a 2,000-mile run across America.

The Nutrimatix Badwater 135

Runners began running the course in the 1970s. The race was formalised in 1987.
2015 saw the most international field in the race's history, with 24 countries represented.
2015 saw 29 women and 68 men sign up, the youngest aged 22, the oldest 80, with an average of 46.
The men's course record is held by Valmir Nunez of Brazil, with a time of 22:51:29 set in 2007.
The women's course record is 26:16:12, set in 2010 by Jamie Donaldson of Littleton.
Along the way are places including Mushroom Rock, Furnace Creek, Salt Creek, Devil's Cornfield, Devil's Golf Course, Stovepipe Wells, Panamint Springs, Keeler, Alabama Hills and Lone Pine.
There is no prize money.

Sir Ranulph Fiennes – 'The world's greatest living explorer'

'I never thought I wouldn't make it.'

Described by the *Guinness Book of Records* as 'the world's greatest living explorer' as long ago as 1984, Sir Ranulph Fiennes has continued to set world records and lead expeditions to the world's remotest regions.

Born in the UK in 1944, just after his father was killed in the Second World War, Fiennes was brought up in South Africa. He returned to the UK to study at Eton College and, after failing his A Levels, joined the Royal Scots Greys (Tanks), with whom he served during the Cold War. Fiennes then joined the SAS (1965–1966), becoming the youngest captain in the British army.

Fiennes' career as an adventurer and explorer began in 1967 with the Jostedalsbreen Glacier Expedition to Norway. Then came the Nile Hovercraft Expedition (1969), the second Jostedalsbreen Glacier Expedition (1970), the Headless Valley Expedition (1971) and the Greenland: Hayes Peninsular Expedition (1976–1978). More recent endeavours have included the Arctic Solo Expedition (2000), Everest Tibet and Everest Nepal summit attempts (2005 and 2008), the north face of the Eiger (2007), Everest Nepal summit (2009) and the 'coldest journey': the Antarctic plateau through polar winter (2014).

But for many he will be remembered as the man who, partnered by friend and medical expert Mike Stroud, completed the first 7x7x7 – seven marathons in seven consecutive days on all seven continents. It was a feat all the more remarkable for the fact that only three and a half months earlier, Fiennes had suffered a massive heart attack, followed by a three-day coma and a double bypass.

The first of the seven marathons was Patagonia at the southern-most tip of Chile. Then came the Falkland Islands followed by Sydney, Australia. On the Wednesday he completed a 26.2-mile run in Singapore. Next came London, then Cairo and finally New York on the Sunday, 183.4 miles in just one week.

Crushed capillaries and stress fractures, torn muscles, cramps and loss of glycogen to fuel a heart working ever harder were among the factors in a schedule which went beyond gruelling. He was also combating dehydration, particularly in Singapore. Another battle was against the effects of jet lag – and all at the age of 59. Stroud and Fiennes were running with a defibrillator to safeguard Fiennes' health.

Fiennes admitted Singapore had almost broken him with its humidity and pollution. 'I hit the pavement and nearly fainted at the end. I felt completely knackered and not able to do another one,' he told the BBC. And yet at the end of it all, Fiennes declared it had been 'good fun'. He completed the New York City Marathon in 5 hours 25 minutes.

And still the feats kept on coming.

In 2015, Fiennes became the oldest Briton to complete the infamous Marathon des Sables at 71 years of age, conquering its 156 miles in six days (5–11 April) in the blistering 50°C (122°F) heat of the Sahara Desert – all in aid of Marie Curie and the charity's work to support people living with a terminal illness.

Immediately after crossing the finishing line, Fiennes explained how touch and go it had been:

> *I don't feel good. My back is bad. Luckily I've had a load of pain killers. Without them it would have been even more difficult. I never thought I*

wouldn't make it. But there were points where I thought the camels, who walk at the rear sweeping up those who are too slow, were getting dangerously close.

The race was not without its victims. With injuries ranging from heart problems to broken legs, 96 people dropped out; but Fiennes made it, and his run brought in more than £134,000 for his chosen charity.

He later reflected:

> *It was particularly bad this year because, as the thirtieth anniversary of the Marathon des Sables, the planners made it the toughest, longest they'd ever made and they did a good job making it very unpleasant. But we did raise lots of money, and it does go towards helping people living with a terminal illness and their loved ones which I reckon from past experiences is worthwhile doing this challenge for.*

In 2010, Sir Ranulph Fiennes was named the UK's top celebrity fundraiser by JustGiving, the UK's most popular online fund-raising platform. Fiennes' expeditions have raised more than £14 million for UK charities.

Sir Ranulph Fiennes: a remarkable record of charity fundraising

1992	£4.2 million	MS Society
1995	£1.6 million	Breakthrough Breast Cancer
2004–2005	£2.3 million	British Heart Foundation
2007–2009	£6.5 million	Marie Curie Cancer Care
2013	$2 million	Seeing is Believing
2013–2015	£2.5 million+	Marie Curie Cancer Care

Nicholas Bourne – The length of Africa, twice

'I wanted more of a challenge in my life.'

UK runner Nicholas Bourne holds the rarest of distinctions. He has twice used muscle power alone to travel the entire length of Africa. First in 1998, he travelled the entire length of Africa from south to north, running all the way, and then, 17 years later, he did the same journey in reverse, this time by bike.

Quite the change of pace for a former international catwalk model.

Bourne's first journey saw him secure a place in the *Guinness Book of Records* by completing the fastest Cape Town to Cairo journey on foot. He ran from South Africa to Egypt in 318 days between 21 January and 5 December 1998, covering more than 7,500 miles and passing through Botswana, Zambia, Tanzania, Kenya, Ethiopia and Sudan.

His original plan was to run from north to south – until Egyptian soldiers stopped his progress at the Sudanese border. Undeterred, Bourne caught a plane to South Africa and completed the route in reverse. Along the way, covering more than 42 miles a day, he wore out 30 pairs of trainers.

Bourne's sister Emma led the backup team as he passed through the heat of the Kalahari Desert and took his chances with the militias of Eastern Africa. On a run dubbed the marathon to end all marathons, he reached altitudes of 12,000 feet, braved deserts, floods and war zones and found himself face to face with a giant cobra, lions and herds of elephants. But in the end, Bourne and his team found their biggest headache was crossing borders.

By the end of it, finishing at the Pyramids in Cairo, he had raised £1 million for the Born Free Foundation and Save the Children.

He told the BBC:

> I wanted more of a challenge in my life [...] I wanted something else in my life. I also wanted to highlight some of the things that I felt were necessary to highlight, about conservation and about education for children.

Seventeen years later, Bourne completed his rare African double, raising funds this time for World Bicycle Relief UK, with a Guinness World Record attempt called Carocap. Bourne and four other cyclists set out from Cairo under the shadow of the

Great Pyramids at Giza on 9 October 2015 – their aim, the fastest crossing of the length of the African continent from Cairo to Cape Town by bicycle.

Their target was to beat Mark Beaumont's record of 41 days 10 hours 22 minutes – and they managed it by four days, covering 6,400 miles in 38 days. Bourne and fellow cyclists Mark Blewett and David Martin reached the finishing line in Cape Town on 15 November. Two others in the team had been forced to pull out ten days before.

Bourne described the challenge as a lot tougher than his 1998 foot-slog, partly because the schedule was shorter and also because they were chasing an existing record. Riding as a team also meant that if a rider was ill or injured, calculations were harder to make in terms of contribution versus time lost. Also adding to the challenge was the fact that 10–12 hours a day in the saddle left very little time to explore or interact with people en route.

Even so, it was a journey packed with unforgettable highlights:

> *Riding at dusk through game parks in Botswana and encountering elephant, lion, giraffe, zebra, buffalo, impala, kudu and oryx just a few metres from where we were riding.*

Back in the UK, Bourne is the man behind the Tour of Wessex, one of the biggest multi-stage cycling races in the world as it winds through quintessentially English countryside along the lanes and byways of the south-west. Each individual stage has its own unique mix of monuments, history and challenging terrain. It is regarded as one of the world's leading cycle events.

Malcolm Attard – On top of the world

*'Your eyes cannot
leave the ground for more
than a couple of seconds.'*

Maltese endurance runner Malcolm Attard has gone both long and high in an impressive running career.

Kenya-based Attard was 37 years old when he pitted his physical and mental stamina against the 2012 Comrades Marathon, proving once again, as so many runners do, that if you are going to push yourself to the limit, you'd better have a good reason for doing so. Declaring his aim to be to 'celebrate mankind's spirit over adversity', Attard was more specifically wanting to support the work of a remarkable Maltese nun, Sister Michelina Micallef, of the Franciscan Sisters of the Heart of Jesus, who has devoted her life to alleviating the lot of those condemned to live in the Nairobi slums.

He rose to the challenge, and with the Comrades safely negotiated, Attard was soon looking for his next adventure. He found it in the highest marathon on earth. The race report concludes: 'The weather was remarkably warm and sunny with no snow this year!' – a sentence which doesn't quite tell the full story. The race in question was the 2013 Everest Marathon.

It was a challenge Attard relished for all the difficulties it brought:

> The terrain is so hazardous that your eyes cannot leave the ground for more than a couple of seconds or you will find yourself lying on the ground with a twisted ankle.

In first place was Nepalese athlete Ram Kumar Raj Bhandari who smashed his own 2011 record in 3:40:43; Bim Bahadur Gurung came second in 3:45:20. Attard was the first non-Nepali runner to finish, completing the course in 5:47:22, to achieve thirteenth place overall.

The race, organised by a company from Worcestershire in the UK, starts at Gorak Shep (5,184 m), just below Everest base camp, and finishes in the Sherpa 'capital' of Namche Bazaar (3,446 m). The route is largely downhill but undulates and also includes steep uphill sections. The race starts at 6.30 a.m. and, with the last 6 miles going out to Thamo and back again, on an exhausting undulating trail, it is essential to finish by nightfall at 6 p.m. Adding to the challenge is the fact the race course is not marked: each runner has to learn the route on the trek up.

In order to acclimatise to the altitude, the international athletes arrive in Nepal two weeks before the race and are joined later by the Nepalese runners. Then under the watchful eyes of a team of medics, the runners begin the long way up, trekking and climbing in freezing temperatures.

Illness is a very real danger. As Attard noted:

> At one point or another we were all struck down by some bug. I was lucky to have fallen ill during the first part of the trek and managed to recover in time to start the race.

And then comes the course itself. The race organisers warn there is likely to be snow and ice at the start, after which competitors will encounter varied terrain. The runners will tackle boulders, grass, sandy scree, stone staircases, trails through forest and exposed paths which contour the mountain sides. Organisers promise the trails will seem quite good to those used to mountain or fell running but warn there are additional hazards by way of narrow suspension bridges and yak trains.

To get their race number, the runners undergo a medical test before the final 5k uphill trek to the start at Gorak Shep. Thereafter for safety's sake, once the race proper is underway, runners must beat the cut-off times at various checkpoints or face elimination. At the end is the satisfaction of knowing that all the funds raised go directly to the Everest Marathon foundation to promote health and education in rural Nepal.

Just as with his run to support the work of Sr Michelina Micallef, Attard found satisfaction in the consequences of his efforts:

> *This is by far one of the toughest races I have ever done but collecting funds to help one of the poorest countries in the world made this challenge even more rewarding.*

CHAPTER TWELVE
AGE SHALL NOT WEARY...

Fauja Singh – Probably the world's oldest marathon runner

'Whatever pain and suffering I've had,
reaped benefits multiple times.'

Plenty of people feel a hundred at the end of a marathon. Fauja Singh was actually a hundred at the start of his. When he completed a Toronto marathon in 2011, Indian-born Singh, who lives in Ilford, Essex, became the world's oldest marathon runner.
  Probably.

His feat was met with a swift intervention from the editor-in-chief at Guinness World Records, Craig Glenday, pointing out it was yet to receive the necessary proof of Singh's actual date of birth.

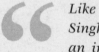 *Like everyone who read about Mr Singh, we were amazed by such an inspirational achievement – to*

finish a marathon at such an old age is awe-inspiring. However, we have yet to receive the documentary evidence that we need to confirm Mr Singh as the world's oldest marathon runner. As much as we'd love to ratify this record, we simply don't have the proof.

And there it still stands. Singh has a British passport that shows his date of birth as 1 April 1911, but it's a birth certificate that the world-record authority requires. Singh possesses a letter from Indian government officials stating that birth records were not kept in 1911, but that's not enough for Guinness. Singh's record cannot officially stand – though the rest of the world is probably happy to let it.

His achievement was to complete the Toronto Waterfront Marathon in 8:25:16. He admits that he hit the wall at 22 miles but pushed on for another two hours and finished in three thousand, eight hundred and fiftieth place, ahead of five other competitors. Singh's coach and interpreter Harmander Singh conveyed the experience for him:

> *Earlier, just before we came around the [final] corner, he said: 'Achieving this will be like getting married again.' He's absolutely overjoyed. He's achieved his lifelong wish.*

Singh was a farmer in the Punjab but moved to Britain in the wake of personal tragedy, taking up running to overcome depression after the deaths of his wife and son. His son's death in 1994 took a particularly hard toll. Singh and his son Kuldip were checking on their fields in the middle of a storm when a piece of corrugated metal, blown by the wind, decapitated Kuldip before his father's eyes. Singh's five other children had emigrated. Left alone, he followed suit, going to live with his youngest son in London where he started attending tournaments organised by the Sikh community. The tournaments included sprinting events, and Singh was drawn in. New friends encouraged him to try long-distance running. When he saw a marathon on television, he decided to give it go.

Singh made his London Marathon debut in 2000 at the age of 89. Between the ages of 89 and 100, Singh, a great-grandfather nicknamed the Turbaned Torpedo, went on to run seven marathons in all, including Frankfurt and Mumbai.

The reasons behind his strength and endurance were never a secret. He always put his stamina down to ginger curry, tea and 'being happy' – and his Toronto run made him exactly that. The day saw him break, unofficially, another eight records for 100-year-old men, his 26.2 miles including all eight distances ranging from 100 m to 5,000 m.

> *The secret to a long and healthy life is to be stress-free. Be grateful for everything you have, stay away from people who are negative, stay smiling and keep running.*

However, even Singh had to concede, at the age of nearly 102, that the time had come to stop. He ran his final race in February 2013, the Hong Kong 10-km race in a time of 1 hour 32 minutes 28 seconds, accompanied by runners from Hong Kong's Sikh community.

In his race retirement, Singh remains physically active, continuing to jog, reaping the benefits of his 14 years of competing. He has also continued to travel. In just a few months, following his final race, he visited Australia, Las Vegas, Dubai, Denmark, Switzerland, France and Luxembourg. Being active is like a medication, he observed – a medication he had no intention of withdrawing.

He told the *Guardian* in October 2013:

> Now I've come to terms with the fact that I don't race any more, I make the best of what I've got. I am still covering distances – although it might take a bit longer now. Running was God's way of distracting me from suffering mentally from the loss of my wife and son. Running took over my time and thoughts. It was God's way of keeping me alive and making me what I am today, and I'm grateful for that. I had no idea I would live this long and would achieve anything. It wasn't a plan.

Bob Dolphin – 500 marathons and counting

'I like the difficulty'

Few runners have shown the dogged determination which has marked Bob Dolphin's running career. Retired entomologist Bob ran his first marathon at the age of 51. He proceeded to run 15-plus marathons a year for the next 26 years, completing his four-hundredth marathon at the age of 77 in 2007. At the age of 82, Bob was gunning for his fifth-hundredth marathon, the twelfth annual

Yakima River Canyon Marathon, a race he directs with his wife, Lenore. One of the race's features is the trademark hug she bestows on him as he crosses the finishing line. Known in the US north-west running community as Team Dolphin, the couple have themselves become a race-day institution, priding themselves on the fun and the friendliness of their home marathon. Dolphin's career high was 24 marathons in 2006.

> *I like the difficulty, the competition in my age class, the sociality among runners, the satisfaction I feel when I complete a race. That's when I feel most of my runner's high – when I can sit down and rest and don't have to count down the miles anymore.*

Considering himself, quite rightly, a runner of advanced years, Dolphin says he runs primarily for the adventure, always training 12 months a year. These days Bob tends to walk his marathons, but looks back fondly on a personal best at the Boston Marathon at the age of 58 when he clocked a time of 3:04:25.

Dolphin has had regular treatments for skin cancers, prostate cancer surgery and hip surgery in late 2004, but has managed to avoid major health setbacks in a running career that started almost by chance, one winter day in the late 1970s in Columbia, Missouri. A blizzard made roads impassable, prompting Bob to walk the 2 miles to his lab. It felt so good that it wasn't long before he moved from walking to running, and from running to running marathons.

It was at a time when running was just beginning to gain widespread popularity, and Dolphin caught the bug. He saw people running in the neighbourhood, and it felt natural to run from home to work. Soon he was running both ways; he lost a few pounds;

but better than that, he discovered he was enjoying it. Bob's first wife died of cancer after a 40-year marriage. In his second wife, Lenore, a non-runner, he found a steadfast supporter and finishing-line volunteer, the perfect companion for his running exploits.

Joy Johnson – A marathoner to the end

'I'll be at the back of the pack, but I don't mind.'

Joy Johnson became the New York City Marathon's oldest woman finisher in 2011 when she clocked a time of 7:44:45 at the age of 84 – a proud moment for the former gym teacher who first took up running when she retired.

After a career teaching high-school physical education in Northern California and with her four children now grown up, Johnson realised she didn't have her own exercise regime. At the age of 59 in 1985, she took a 3-mile walk with her husband, found it energising and soon started jogging. The enjoyment deepened, and within a few years she was a fixture at local road races.

Raised on a Minnesota dairy farm, Johnson went on to run an average of three marathons a year, which she backed up with dozens of shorter races. She would always run with a bow in her hair, a trademark which became ever more recognised as her fame started to spread. After her husband's death, her daily routine was fixed: rising at 4 a.m., she would breakfast on coffee and oatmeal, read the Bible and then head off for a run on the track at the school where she once taught.

Sadly, running lost an inspirational figure in November 2013, when Johnson died the day after completing her twenty-fifth New York City Marathon. She was the day's oldest finisher.

Johnson, from San Jose, California, apparently fell and hit her head around the marathon's 20-mile mark. Medical staff wanted to take her straight to hospital, but Joy insisted on finishing the course, which she duly did in 7:57:41, head bloodied but spirit utterly unbroken. 'I wasn't watching where I was going,' she told her sister shortly after finishing. 'It looks just awful, but I'm fine.' Her rule for any race was to make sure she always smiled down the home straight, and she managed it, among the very last of the day's 50,266 finishers.

Johnson was still smiling the next morning at a post-marathon reception, but sadly her injuries caught up with her just hours later. Her obituary in the *New York Times Magazine* recorded:

> *Afterward, back in her Midtown hotel room, she removed her medal and lay down for a nap. Finally finished, she drifted off to sleep, never regaining consciousness. She died later that day.*

Just the day before her final race, Johnson said: 'I always say I'm going to run until I drop. I'm going to die in my tennis shoes. I just don't know when I'm going to quit.' The *New York Times Magazine* labelled her 'a marathoner to the end'. *TODAY News* offered a similarly touching obituary: 'She was a winner, a relentless competitor, and as befits her name, a pleasure to be around.'

Johnson's thoughts and achievements were preserved for posterity in a poignant documentary made by ESPN. The programme, titled *Every Day,* began by showing Johnson reading her favourite passage from the Bible, a passage she used to read every morning as the best possible start to every new day.

> *But they that wait upon the Lord shall renew their strength; they shall mount up with wings as eagles; they shall run, and not be weary; and they shall walk, and not faint.*

Louise Rossetti – Overcoming personal tragedy

'It's a release. I just like to run. You forget everything, noticing the flowers or somebody is putting on a new porch, or whatever.'

The frustration of running around a race track was all the inspiration Louise Rossetti needed when she took an exercise class at the age of 50 in 1971. 'Gee, can't we go outside and run?' she complained, and off she went, off the leash at the start of an inspirational running career which she chronicled race by race in lovingly compiled scrapbooks.

The oldest of nine children, Louise Bernazani was born in Boston where she went to business school. She married Peter Rossetti in 1945 and settled in Saugus, where he started an insurance company two years later. By the early 1970s, she was craving exercise. Running proved the answer.

Rossetti's first race was a 5-miler in May 1971 when she tied for last place. Thousands more races followed, each one meticulously documented in her scrapbooks with race numbers, notes about the weather and newspaper cuttings all appended.

Sadly, Rossetti's running was soon to merge with personal tragedy. When her younger daughter, Suzanne, was murdered in Arizona in 1981, Rossetti's response was to race all the more. The Rossettis became involved in a national programme for parents of murdered children. For Rossetti, running was the outlet, but not necessarily an escape from the tragedy. Her son Peter Jnr remarked that running for his mother was her way of communicating with Suzanne.

Running and commemoration converged when Louise launched an annual 5k race, with the proceeds going to a scholarship fund in her daughter's name. When her husband died in 1993, Rossetti's response, once again, was to race even more.

Rossetti freely admitted she was never going to threaten the race leaders, but as the *Boston Globe* noted in her obituary, she firmly established herself as 'an institution in Boston running circles, someone who was more inspirational at the back of the pack than those breaking the finish line tape'.

Rossetti belonged to at least eight running clubs, and a highlight came in 2001, the year she turned 80, when she competed in 164 races, sometimes competing in two on the same day. She capped the year in December 2001 by carrying the Olympic torch for one leg of the relay on its route to Salt Lake City.

> *I think runners are a great breed of people. They treat me like a queen. I'm embarrassed, really, by all the attention they shower upon me.*

Rossetti starred in the independent film *Run Grammie Run* about an elderly woman training for a marathon, but it was for her own running that she will be remembered.

The twenty-second Annual Louise Rossetti Women's 5k went ahead on Wednesday, 17 June 2015 as the first anniversary of her death approached. 'Please come and remember your past memories of Louise,' the race organisers urged. Many people did – and did so with huge affection.

Sister Madonna Buder – The Iron Nun

*'I love the feeling
I get when I whizz past
people younger than me
and they say, "I want to be like
you when I get to your age!"'*

Somehow you wouldn't expect the current world record holder for the oldest person ever to finish an Ironman triathlon to be a nun. But Sister Madonna Buder (*b.* 1930) is no ordinary nun. She is the Iron Nun.

The Ironman triathlon consists of a 2.4-mile swim, 112-mile bike ride and a full-marathon 26.2-mile run. The Iron Nun has no fewer than 45 Ironmans among more than 340 completed triathlons.

Sister Buder was 14 when she decided she wanted to be a nun. The running didn't come until much later. At the age of 23, she entered the Sisters of the Good Shepherd convent in St Louis where she remained until 1990 when she changed orders and was sent to Spokane, Washington, to serve with the Sisters for Christian Community.

She started running at the age of 48 when she was told it would be good for mind and body. Racing soon followed. Accepting the public probably wasn't used to racing nuns, she checked first with the bishop. As she told *Cosmopolitan* in 2014, his response was simple and direct: 'Sister, I wish some of my priests would do what you're doing!'

Sister Buder was inspired to join running clubs, and soon the triathlon challenge started to beckon. She completed her first at the age of 52 in 1982, in Banbridge, Ireland.

> *I felt an immense amount of accomplishment after I finished that race; I was content.*

But she was not content to leave it there. More and more triathlons followed. Buder earned the title 'Iron Nun' when she became the oldest woman ever to complete the Hawaii Ironman in 2005 at the age of 75.

Inevitably, Sister Buder detects the hand of a higher authority in her achievements and adventures, not least when an eerie omen seemed to foretell the ghastly bombing at the 2013 Boston Marathon in which she was competing. On the morning before the race, a police officer gave her his card and told her to call him if she needed help; a young boy nearby urged her to memorise the number on the card. She did so – and, amid the chaos later that day, she phoned it. Sister Buder was just approaching the twenty-first mile when the bombers struck. The officer duly escorted her from the scene.

She was spared the carnage – blessed to carry on boogying.

> *People often ask me how I train for these kinds of arduous events, and to that I say, 'I just boogie.' My training is very functional. I run to church every day if the weather permits. I'll bike 40 miles to swim in a lake near my house and on the weekends I'll go for a longer run. I also try to run to the jail when it's nice out to talk to the inmates about Jesus and read scriptures to them. I always come back home feeling so blessed.*

Sab Koide – Cab fare not needed

'The most uplifting part is to get to the 26 miles. I try to race the last two-tenths of a mile to show I'm still in good shape.'

Sab Koide of Dobbs Ferry, New York began running at the age of 56. By his eighty-fifth birthday, he had completed 60 marathons, 28 of them in New York City – no mean achievement for a man who was happy to label himself an accidental marathoner.

As he has passed through the decades, so the numbers in his age category have inevitably dwindled. Standing at the start of the 2004 New York City Marathon, Koide was one of just four in the over-80s category. But he remained undaunted.

At the start of his running career, Koide admitted that running seemed to him 'like being on a treadmill, expending energy but really going nowhere and getting exhausted along the way'. In 1976, his wife, Sumi, gave his running precisely the focus it needed. Sumi, a retired professor of medicine at the Albert Einstein College of Medicine, organised a 3-mile charity road race and signed up her husband and two sons.

It wasn't long before Sab discovered a natural talent – and a way to control slightly high blood pressure. He entered the New York City Marathon the following year – much to his wife's concern. She sent him off with a note: 'If you have found him fallen on the street, please take him to New York Hospital. Here is $20 for a cab.'

She needn't have worried. He has been running ever since.

With a degree in internal medicine and a PhD in biochemistry, Koide worked in research at Rockefeller University until his retirement. He runs 40 miles a week in the six weeks leading up to marathons – all after a rather undignified start to his competitive career. Koide ran his first marathon as an unregistered runner and was forced out by a race official as he approached the finishing line. He later joked that at his age, it was his privilege to admit to such transgressions.

Koide was among the runners as New York City tried to get itself back on its feet after the devastation wrought by Hurricane Sandy in 2012. The charity God's Love We Deliver was among those leading the way with its fundraising Race to Deliver running event. In the aftermath of the hurricane, its work was even more crucial than ever, with the charity stretched to the limit. After delivering more than 8,000 meals to people displaced by the storm, God's Love found itself racing to restock its shelves for the coming holiday season. The 2012 Race to Deliver event in Central Park needed a bumper turnout and got it, attracting athletes of all abilities. Among them was 89-year-old Koide, who finished arm in arm with New York Road Runners president and CEO Mary Wittenberg.

Over the years, his exploits have proved more than enough to secure his place in the official list of Dobbs Ferry Notable People.

Gladys Burrill and Harriette Thompson – The world's oldest female marathoners

'Perseverance, strength, courage...
you just have to keep going.'

Born in the month the First World War ended, Gladys Burrill – known as the Gladyator – became the oldest woman to complete a marathon when she passed the finishing line in the Honolulu Marathon in Hawaii on 12 December 2010.

At the age of 92 years 19 days, great-grandmother Burrill power-walked and jogged her way around the course to beat the previous record held by Jenny Wood-Allen, a Scot who completed the London Marathon at the age of 90 in 2002.

The achievement was simply the latest in a busy life.

The youngest of six children of Finnish immigrants, Burrill lost her father on her second birthday. She now divides her time between Oregon and Honolulu, a far cry from the Washington state farm where her mother brought up the family alone. Life was hard, particularly at the age of 11 when Burrill contracted polio. She later recovered. Always, she said, a healthy lifestyle was key to happiness and to overcoming difficulties.

> *Sometimes I go out [walking] with the weight of the world on my shoulders and come back feeling so strong and renewed.*

Burrill had been an aircraft pilot, mountain climber, desert hiker and horseback rider before running her first marathon in 2004 at the age of 86.

Training simply by regularly walking 30 to 50 miles a week, Burrill went on to complete five out of seven Honolulu Marathons, missing out in 2008 and 2009. In 2008, just days after the death of her husband, Burrill said it was stress and grief that caused her to end her marathon just 1 mile short of the finishing line. In 2009, a stomach problem put her out at mile 16. But in 2010 she was back for the record. She later said the difference was that she felt much more at peace. Indeed, she would have been 2 minutes quicker had she not stopped to pray a couple of hundred metres from the finishing line.

A Seventh-day Adventist, Burrill was joined on the course by her son and grandson at different points. Jim Barahal, president of the Honolulu Marathon, declared himself astonished at Burrill's feat:

> *I think it is absolutely unbelievable. It is inspirational [...] to anyone who has an elderly parent or perhaps has lost someone to realise what she is doing at her age. It is just astonishing. What an inspiration.*

Barahal later inducted Burrill into the marathon's Hall of Fame. The plaque says the woman known as 'the Gladyator' 'redefines what is possible'. It hails her as 'a true inspiration not only to the people of Hawaii but to people around the world'. State governor Neil Abercrombie also honoured Burrill at the ceremony, presenting her a proclamation designating the day as Gladys Burrill Day in Hawaii.

Following Honolulu 2010, Burrill announced she was retiring from the marathon distance.

For Burrill, who has 18 grandchildren and 26 great-grandchildren, it was only ever really a question of getting out there and enjoying the outdoor life, she told NBC News:

> *Just get out there and walk or run. I like walking because you can stop and smell the roses, but it's a rarity that I stop. It's so important to think positive. It's easy to get discouraged and be negative. It makes such a difference in how you feel and your outlook on everything.*

Burrill's record stood until 2015 when cancer survivor Harriette Thompson completed San Diego's Rock 'n' Roll Marathon in 7:24:36 at the age of 92 years and 65 days. A classically trained pianist, Thompson, from Charlotte, North Carolina, mentally plays piano songs in her head as she runs, to help her get through the long-distance races.

She started marathon running when she was 76 years old and went on to raise more than $100,000 for America's Leukemia and Lymphoma Society. Thompson watched both her parents and three brothers die of cancer; her husband of 67 years also died of cancer. A member of her church asked her to sponsor a marathon runner in aid of cancer research. Thompson's response was to run one herself. Initially she planned to walk, but when she saw everyone else running, she simply joined in.

Thompson went on to complete San Diego's Rock 'n' Roll Marathon 16 times in the next 18 years, each time on behalf of the Leukemia and Lymphoma Society and Team in Training. Because of its dedication to the Leukemia and Lymphoma Society, it's the only marathon she has ever run.

Thompson has also fought her own battles against cancer. In 2010, 2011 and 2012, she ran the marathon while fighting oral cancer; in 2013, she missed it because of surgery. She returned in 2014 and almost matched her time in 2015, her record-breaking year.

The race organisers flew her to San Diego first class, chauffeured her around the city and used her as part of their *Why Running Rocks* campaign. For the race itself, Thompson wore white tights to conceal bandages on her legs to cover wounds from radiation treatment; and she admits there were times she nearly didn't make it. A hill at 21 miles felt more like a mountain, and she found herself thinking, 'This is sort of crazy at my age.'

But as she came down the hill, her energy returned. Her son Brenny kept her topped up on carbohydrates; and her thoughts turned to her fundraising for cancer research and all the people it touched.

 I don't think I'd be living today if I didn't do this running. I'm helping them and they're kind of helping me.

CHAPTER THIRTEEN
THE MODERN GREATS

Catherine Ndereba – Catherine the Great

'Something was in my blood.'

Described by the *Chicago Tribune* in 2008 as 'the greatest women's marathoner of all time', Catherine Ndereba is more generally referred to as Catherine the Great.

Born Wincatherine Nyambura Ndereba in Nyeri County, Kenya in 1972, she began running at school and just kept on going. She would creep out of the dorm every morning and run; at night, she would just about make it back in time for dinner. Her schoolmates didn't understand. They teased 'Crazy Ndereba', as they called her: 'Some were runners, and not even they were able to understand what I loved. Something was in my blood. I could not part with it.'

Ndereba recalls it came instinctively:

> " *I would always run. I started running at school, and I didn't know that anyone would run anywhere else. So after school, I was just running on trails as I didn't know about cross-country or track. When I was at school I didn't know that there would be coaches for running. I just used to wake up and did my running. I did not know what I was doing. I didn't know that you were supposed to stretch if you want to run well. A lot of stuff. But keeping on running and running and running made me a good athlete anyway.*

Fortunately, there was family support. Her brother, Samuel, and sister, Anastasia, who were brought up with her on the south-western slopes of Mount Kenya, also ran marathons. There was also job security. Runners in Kenya are often employed by the government, but are expected to work for a government service. Ndereba joined the Kenya Prisons College to train to become a prison guard. There she met her future husband, Anthony, who remained a prison guard throughout her glittering running career.

As soon as Ndereba started training in earnest, it was clear she was going to be something special, beating fellow runners with ease. She ran for Kenya for the first time in Seoul in 1995. Named Road Runner of the Year by *Runner's World* in 1996 and 1998, she broke world records for the 5-km, 12-km, 15-km and 10-mile distances, but it was to be in the marathon that she achieved her greatest results.

Ndereba won the Boston Marathon four times (2000, 2001, 2004 and 2005), running successively, 2:26:11, 2:23:53, 2:24:27 and 2:25:12. In 2001, she ran 2:18:47 in the Chicago Marathon to break the women's marathon world record, a record she held until Paula Radcliffe broke it a year later with 2:17:18 on the same course. Named Athlete of the Year by the IAAF in 2001, Ndereba went on to win silver medals in the marathon in the 2004 Athens Olympics and in the 2008 Beijing Olympics.

Career highlights

2008 Beijing Olympics	Silver
2007 World Championships	Gold
2005 World Championships	Gold
2004 Athens Olympics	Silver
2003 World Championships	Gold

Tegla Loroupe – Championing peace and social change

'I want to show that women don't need to feel like useless people.'

Tegla Loroupe's victory in the 1994 New York City Marathon went far beyond the personal. It inspired a continent. Kenyan men had been winning marathons for years. Loroupe was the first African woman to win a major marathon. She returned to New York City the following year and won it again. Since then, Kenyan women have been at the top of the sport. Her achievement wasn't simply about 26.2 miles; it was about social change. As the New York Road Runners' elite athlete recruiter David Monti told the *Wall Street Journal* in 2013: 'Tegla Loroupe changed the sport of distance running radically by inspiring African women to get in the game.'

Loroupe was born in 1973 in remote western Kenya and raised on a farm in the village of Kapsait, about 200 miles north-west of Nairobi. Effectively she started training by running 6 miles to and from school as a barefoot 6-year-old, but both her running and her education brought her into conflict with her family. Her father considered schools and running to be a waste of time for a woman. Tradition dictated that her role was domestic.

But Loroupe rebelled, drawing her inspiration as she grew older from the Norwegian runner Ingrid Kristiansen. 'Women always have to fight. Nothing is easy for us,' Loroupe later said. With her older sister, Albina, secretly supporting her, Loroupe started to compete and began to train with the Kenyan men.

Loroupe was fortunate to step up her running at a time when the New York City Marathon had identified Kenyan women runners as an untapped resource. She was deemed too young at 20 years old to run the 1993 New York City Marathon, but in 1994, she came of age on the course. She ran it and won it in a time of 2:27:37. She then made it two in two when she won it again in 1995, running 2:28:06. Her achievement was particularly incredible, as Albina died in sudden, tragic circumstances just days before the race. Back home in Kenya, she was hailed as an inspiration for all African women. Things were changing.

Between 1997 and 1999, Loroupe won three consecutive world half-marathon championships. She was also the world's fastest female marathoner, a title she held from 19 April 1998–30 September 2001. She took the record with a time of 2:20:47 in the 1998 Rotterdam Marathon and then broke her own record with a time of 2:20:43 in the 1999 Berlin Marathon.

Inevitably, Loroupe was one of the favourites at the 2000 Sydney Olympics, both for the marathon and the 10,000 m – until a bout of food poisoning left her struggling. Loroupe battled to thirteenth place in the marathon and, the next day, managed to secure fifth place in the 10,000 m. She said she felt compelled to run by the thought of all the people looking up to her back home. Other marathon victories came in London and Rome in 2000 and Lausanne in 2002. She also held world records at 1 hour and at the distances 20, 25 and 30 km.

Arguably she became even more of an icon when she stepped down from marathon running to run, instead, a foundation for peace, back home in north-west Kenya in an area where tribes have been warring for centuries. Battles rage for days, schools are forced to close and families are displaced. Loroupe responded by setting up the Tegla Loroupe Peace Foundation, which runs a number of conflict resolution programmes.

In 2006, she also founded the 10k Peace Race, which pitted 2,000 warriors from six different tribes against each other in non-violent competition. Aiming to foster friendship between the warring communities on the Kenyan–Ugandan border, the peace race targets mainly young people. Its impact, socially and politically, was recognised when it was endorsed by the IAAF's Athletics for a Better World programme, an initiative that promotes projects which use athletics as a tool for social good.

> *I grew up in a pastoral environment where life was really hard because of the local conflicts between the tribes and people stealing cattle. All of this on top of conditions that were hard to start with. I*

was lucky. I had talent and was able to make a success out of running and I felt that I wanted to give things back to the community I grew up in.

In 2006, Loroupe was named a United Nations Ambassador of Sport. She is also a member of Champions for Peace, a group of athletes seeking to use the power of sport to bring an end to conflict.

Tegla Loroupe's achievements

1993 World Championships, 10,000 m	4th
1994 New York City Marathon	1st
1995 Boston Marathon	9th
1995 New York City Marathon	1st
1995 World Championships, 10,000 m	3rd
1996 Boston Marathon	2nd
1996 New York City Marathon	7th
1996 Olympic Games, 10,000 m	6th
1997 Half-marathon World Championships	1st
1997 New York City Marathon	7th
1997 Rotterdam Marathon	1st
1998 Goodwill Games, 10,000 m	1st
1998 Half-marathon World Championships	1st

1998 New York City	3rd
1998 Rotterdam Marathon	1st
1999 Berlin Marathon	1st
1999 World Championships, 10,000 m	3rd
1999 Half-marathon World Championships	1st
2000 Kenyan National Championships, 10,000 m	1st
2000 London Marathon	1st
2002 Lausanne Marathon	1st

Paula Radcliffe – Still no one else is coming close

'It was just a matter of keeping my head strong.'

The true measure of Paula Radcliffe's greatness is the fact that her record still stands comprehensively unchallenged 13 years after she set it.

In the years 2003–2016, the fastest time for a men's marathon has been broken six times as it moves ever closer to breaking that tantalising, much-fabled 2-hour mark. Khalid Khannouchi's record of 2:05:38 set on 14 April 2002 has been replaced in those years by Dennis Kimetto's 2:02:57, set on 28 September 2014, and you sense it won't be too long before Kimetto's record is broken in turn. In fact, it was nearly broken in the 2016 London Marathon. And yet Paula Radcliffe's women's record of 2:15:25, set at the age of 29 in the 2003 London Marathon, still stands supreme.

And just to underline that supremacy, it has to be remembered that it was Radcliffe's own record that she broke, clocking in at 2:17:18 in Chicago in 2002. It took the men a dozen years to knock two and a half minutes off their record time. It took Radcliffe six months.

Radcliffe told the *Guardian* in 2013:

> *Looking back you think, 'Oh actually that was a really big deal at the time.' But I was so ready to run that and believed that was what I'd do that day that it wasn't a massive big shock or a surprise. From the start we all said we mustn't set a limit on it. That was our motto at the time: no limits.*

More than 13 years after that London record, Radcliffe still holds first and second position in the world record tables. In fact, if you look at the list of the fastest women's marathons ever run – as opposed to a list of just those that broke the previously held record – Radcliffe occupies the top three slots, plus sixth for good measure.

In 2012, 16 men ran faster than Khannouchi's 2002 record; the year's fastest woman was Mary Keitany with 2:18:37, more than 3 minutes slower than Radcliffe's record.

The more you look at it the more remarkable Radcliffe's achievement appears. No one else is coming close, and in some ways the gap seems to be getting bigger. Women can now win major marathons without having to break the 2-hour 20-minute mark. Predicting world record performances is never a very good idea, but it seems likely Radcliffe's record will stand for a good few more years yet, as Deena Kastor, holder of the American record at 2:19:36, suggests:

> *Records are meant to be broken, but I am confident we will continue to see Paula's record in the books for decades longer. Fans of this sport will continue viewing her [2-hour 15-minute] performance as iconic, heroic and a stunning sprint of 26.2 miles.*

Blocking out the pain by counting to a hundred again and again, Radcliffe maintained an unrelenting pace in London 2003, running the twenty-fourth mile in five minutes and three seconds, and the twenty-fifth mile in five minutes and eight seconds. It was a phenomenal run.

Much has been written on why Radcliffe is so far ahead. The presence of pacemakers, her running economy, her mental approach, her remarkable pain threshold and her emphasis on running a negative split are just some of the factors that are pored over. But the best, most comprehensive answer is that she was, quite simply, an extraordinary athlete.

As the men still chase that 2-hour mark, the thinking increasingly seems to be that we have already seen its equivalent for the women, in Radcliffe's astonishing 2003 London run – a woman from Cheshire standing alone in a sport dominated by East Africans. Her time would have won every men's Olympic marathon until 1960.

In 1964, when Britain's Basil Heatley held the men's world record and Dale Greig the women's, the difference between the sexes was 1 hour 14 minutes. Radcliffe's London run made the gap between the men's and women's marathon record the closest it had ever been, just over 10 minutes. The gap has now slipped back to just over 13 minutes.

Hugh Brasher, London Marathon race director, recalls Radcliffe's 2003 run as the day women's marathon running changed forever:

> *It heralded a boom in women's running that has carried on since. Immediately sales of women's running shoes increased dramatically, even to the extent that the most popular models were sold out for months. Suddenly Paula had made it acceptable for women to be out running in the streets. She started a women's running revolution.*

Radcliffe's popularity is reflected in the way Britain shared her disappointments every bit as much as it shared her triumphs. She consistently provided iconic marathon moments, although not all of them were happy ones. Radcliffe failed to place at the 2004 Olympic Games in Athens, a disappointment followed by tearful interviews in which we all felt her pain. Typically, she roared back to win the New York Marathon later that year and then won gold in the women's marathon at the 2005 World Championships in Helsinki. But Olympic success was always to elude her. After suffering a muscle cramp in the 2008 Olympic Games in Beijing, she finished in twenty-third place. Completing a trio of Olympic heartbreaks, she withdrew from the 2012 Olympics in London.

Her final years in the sport were dogged by injury. She certainly admits to frustration that it became ever more difficult to repeat her successes. In an interview, she recalled going back to her training base in Albuquerque in 2005, 2007 and 2008 and failing to get close to the 10-mile tempo run she was doing in 2003.

> *At the time you think you're going to keep on improving. Until then, every time I'd gone there I'd taken the time down further. Then you suddenly*

think, 'I'm not going to be able to get back to that.' I used to get really frustrated and stressed, trying to push myself to it.

Radcliffe knew her career was coming to a close. Fortunately the fates conspired to give her exactly the send-off she deserved when she ran her final London Marathon in 2015 in front of a crowd that roared her on every step of the way. Running to say farewell rather than to compete, her London run brought an ecstatic ovation for the champion of champions.

Radcliffe was six times world champion (Marathon 2005, World Cross 2001 and 2002, World Half-marathon 2000, 2001 and 2003) and seven times a big-city marathon winner (London three times, New York three times and Chicago once). In her final marathon, she was given the fond farewell she deserved.

> *Down the last mile I thought, 'I don't care about the time.' I just wanted to thank as many people as I could. I knew it would be emotional and it was so emotional. I nearly lost it at Birdcage Walk but the crowds bowled me over. I wanted it to last forever.*

Women's world record marathon progression

1964	Dale Greig (GBR)	3:27:45
1971	Elizabeth Bonner (USA)	2:55:22
1981	Joyce Smith (GBR)	2:29:57

1985	Ingrid Kristiansen (NOR)	2:21:06
2001	Catherine Ndereba (KEN)	2:18:47
2003	Paula Radcliffe (GBR)	2:15:25

Mary Keitany – The power of motherhood

'The weariness that builds up looking after
your family is weaker than the inner strength
that your children will give you.'

Some runners are motivated by wanting to be the best; others might even admit that the money makes them quicken their step. Mary Keitany, one of the most formidable female marathoners of recent years and officially the second-fastest woman in history, says it is motherhood that drives her forward.

As she told the *New York City Marathon* website:

> *Maternity is a fantastic experience that changes your life. It makes you more responsible and mature. The new attitude also reflects on the dedication you put into training because you realise you are not just running for money or for glory, but for giving your children a better future by improving your performances.*

Keitany became a mother for the first time with the birth of Jared in June 2008 and for a second time with her daughter, Samantha, in April 2013. For each she took a year out, stopping in the third month of pregnancy and resuming when the children were six months old. She insists she didn't regret a moment.

> **Becoming a mother is the most important thing that happened in my life, I don't regret having given up on some races in order to accomplish this. I cannot say if these years that I have missed would have made my legs stronger than now, but I can guarantee that without maternity I wouldn't have the same motivation that I have now. This motivation pushes me and makes me train hard; it makes me want to improve myself day by day.**

Born in Kenya in 1982, Keitany became world half-marathon champion in 2009. Mary Wittenberg, director of the New York City Marathon, suggested she should step up to the full marathon distance. She did so in the 2010 NYC Marathon, finishing third in 2:29:01. In the meantime, she remained dominant in the half-marathon, smashing the women's record when she won the Ras Al Khaimah Half-marathon in 2011 in 1:05:50.

Keitany returned to the full marathon distance in 2011 and did so gloriously when she won the London Marathon in a time of 2:19:19, a time she bettered when she successfully defended her title the following year, at the age of 30, with a time of 2:18:37. Only Paula Radcliffe has run faster, three times.

In 2012, watchers were quick to latch on to the huge potential she showed in the five-minute mile she ran between the twenty-third and twenty-fourth mile. It fuelled hope for an Olympic gold in London that August. In the event, she fell behind to finish a disappointing fourth.

Motherhood was the theme of 2013 before Keitany returned in spectacular fashion in 2014 for the first of two of the greatest successes in her career, winning the New York City Marathon in 2:25:07 – 'Definitely the most thrilling day of my life,' she later said.

Keitany was back again in New York in 2015 for a race in which she played a waiting game. She waited and then made her move. Keitany ran the twenty-first mile in 5 minutes 14 seconds, the twenty-second mile in 5 minutes 13 seconds, and the twenty-third in 5 minutes 16 seconds – enough to blow her competitors away. She crossed the line in 2:24:25 to become the first woman successfully to defend her title in the New York City Marathon since Paula Radcliffe won in 2007 and 2008.

> *I learned lessons here in 2011, so today I had to be patient and wait. I was very confident coming here. At home my training was perfect and I was coming to defend my title. It helped that I understood the course, as the field was very tough.*

Experience was crucial; motherhood did the rest.

Fastest ever women's marathon times

1	Paula Radcliffe (GBR)	London	1st	13 April 2003	2:15:25
2	Paula Radcliffe (GBR)	Chicago	1st	13 October 2002	2:17:18
3	Paula Radcliffe (GBR)	London	1st	17 April 2005	2:17:42
4	Liliya Shobukhova (RUS)	Chicago	1st	9 October 2011 *	2:18:20

5	Mary Keitany (KEN)	London	1st	22 April 2012	2:18:37
6	Catherine Ndereba (KEN)	Chicago	1st	7 October 2001	2:18:47
7	Paula Radcliffe (GBR)	London	1st	14 April 2002	2:18:56
8	Rita Sitienei Jeptoo (KEN)	Boston	1st	21 April 2014	2:18:57
9	Tiki Gelana (ETH)	Rotterdam	1st	15 April 2012	2:18:58
10	Mizuki Noguchi (JPN)	Berlin	1st	25 September 2005	2:19:12
11	Irina Mikitenko (GER)	Berlin	1st	28 September 2008	2:19:19
12	Mary Keitany (KEN)	London	1st	17 April 2011	2:19:19
13	Gladys Cherono (KEN)	Berlin	1st	27 September 2015	2:19:25
14	Catherine Ndereba (KEN)	Chicago	2nd	13 October 2002	2:19:26
15	Aselefech Mergia (ETH)	Dubai	1st	27 January 2012	2:19:31
16	Lucy Kabuu (KEN)	Dubai	2nd	27 January 2012	2:19:34
17	Deena Kastor (USA)	London	1st	23 April 2006	2:19:36
18	Yingjie Sun (CHN)	Beijing	1st	19 October 2003	2:19:39
19	Yoko Shibui (JPN)	Berlin	1st	26 September 2004	2:19:41
20	Florence Kiplagat (KEN)	Berlin	1st	25 September 2011	2:19:44

* Shobukhova's time was erased when she was disqualified because of 'biological passport abnormalities'

Geoffrey Mutai – The world record that wasn't

*'I see this as a gift from God. I don't
have more words to add.'*

Even with the quest for the elusive first-ever 2-hour marathon gathering pace, you wouldn't expect a marathon runner to knock nearly a minute off the world record in one go.

However, the Kenyan Geoffrey Mutai did exactly that in the 2011 Boston Marathon, running 2:03:02 to smash Haile Gebrselassie's record of 2:03:59 (Berlin, 2008). Mutai's time was the fastest marathon ever run at that point. But it didn't count as a world record, and nor was it ever going to.

The Boston course is not deemed to be record-eligible by the IAAF. Their rules state that a course's start and finish points cannot be farther apart than 50 per cent of the race distance. The Boston Marathon starts 26.2 miles from the finish. The course also exceeds the overall decrease in elevation permitted from start to finish, so it is therefore doubly disqualified.

But whatever the record books say, there was no taking away from Mutai's remarkable run, a new course record knocking nearly 3 minutes off the previous standard which had been set the year before. Twenty-nine-year-old Mutai pulled away from Moses Mosop in the final 250 m. Mosop's consolation was running the then second-fastest marathon ever in his first competitive marathon. Tom Grilk, the executive director of the Boston Athletic Association, hailed Mutai's performance as a once-in-a-lifetime moment: 'No one could have predicted that a time like that would be run.'

For Mutai, who comes from the Koibatek region of Kenya, between Eldoret and Nairobi in the Great Rift Valley province, it was a remarkable comeback. Nine years before, he'd decided to quit running because of injury.

The oldest of nine children, Mutai started competitive running at the age of 12. When Mutai's father lost his job at a textile company in Eldoret, Mutai was unable to move up to secondary school. He had to earn a living and turned to running. Mutai progressed to the 3,000 m steeplechase event, but when he injured his Achilles tendon, he decided to stop running completely and find a job. It seemed his running career was over at the age of 21. However, he later lost his job and returned to running again. His misfortune proved athletics' gain.

Mutai remains self-coached:

> *I have a training programme that is unique and caters for many distances. That is why I prefer to train on my own without any coach since it is easier for me to adjust for the race I'm running next.*

In 2011, Mutai won the New York City Marathon, setting a course record of 2:05:06, and returned to retain his title with a 2:08:24 run in the Big Apple in 2013 when the marathon resumed after the 2012 cancellation in the aftermath of Hurricane Sandy. In between times, in 2012, Mutai crossed the line to win the thirty-ninth Berlin Marathon ahead of his compatriot Dennis Kimetto.

In 2014, he came sixth in both the London and New York City Marathons.

Personal bests

10,000 m	27:27.79 Nairobi	26 June 2010
10 km	27:19 Boston	26 June 2011
15 km	42:15 Ras Al Khaimah	15 February 2013
20 km	56:05 Ras Al Khaimah	15 February 2013
Half-marathon	58:58 Ras Al Khaimah	15 February 2013
25 km	1:13:25 Berlin	27 September 2015
30 km	1:28:11 Berlin	30 September 2012
Marathon	2:04:15 Berlin	30 September 2012

Kenenisa Bekele – A stunning marathon debut

'What do I tell you? Everything is a challenge. That's how we are made in Ethiopia. It's through a struggle.'

The race is far from run for Ethiopia's Kenenisa Bekele, one of the rising stars of marathon racing.

Growing up admiring Ethiopian Olympic gold medal-winning runners Haile Gebrselassie, Fatuma Roba and Derartu Tulu, Bekele (*b*. 1982) took ninth place in 1999 in the junior race at the world cross-country championships and took the silver medal in the 3,000 m at the IAAF's world youth championship. He went on to set a record for the most career wins in the history of the world cross-country championships, with a remarkable 11 titles to his name.

In 2003, Bekele started to show what he could do on a track, going on to win Olympic gold medals in the 10,000 m in 2004 and in both the 5,000 m and the 10,000 m in 2008.

And then came his marathon debut.

For a while it seemed he might be going head to head with Mo Farah in London in 2014. It was a juicy prospect, a chance for revenge in a way. Bekele had reigned supreme over the 5,000 m and 10,000 m on the world and Olympic stage until Farah claimed his crowns. But the London battle didn't materialise. Bekele was unable to agree financial terms with the organisers. Paris and London offered the same terms. Bekele opted for Paris, the week before, as the gentler introduction to the distance. It was no to London.

> *There are very strong competitors there, tougher maybe than Paris, and I wanted to run an even pace. It was very important for me to win on my debut as well, and maybe London is more difficult for that.*

His result suggested he had made exactly the right decision. Bekele stormed home to win the 2014 Paris Marathon, crossing the line in 2:05:04 to shave 8 seconds off the course record which had been set two years earlier by Kenyan Stanley Biwott. Bekele's time, which came with almost 2 minutes in hand over second place, was the sixth-fastest marathon debut in history on a record-eligible course. It was also the fastest ever debut by someone older than 30. He labelled the result 'very positive', speculating, 'I think in the future I'll do better.'

Disappointment followed Bekele's Paris triumph, however. He finished a below-expectations fourth with 2:05:51 in the 2014 Chicago Marathon, and then in the Dubai Marathon in January 2015, he dropped out of the race after 18 miles, citing pain in both hamstrings. He then withdrew from the London Marathon in April 2015.

But there is no doubt that Bekele remains a strong marathon contender. Speaking before his Dubai trip in 2015, he felt he was learning the lessons that the marathon insists you learn. Experience was to be his new weapon.

> I've learned from my races in Paris and Chicago. Coming to the marathon, you race with the distance itself. It doesn't matter if there are strong competitors or not. In a marathon, anything can challenge you. Even the distance itself can challenge you, because it's not like 5,000, 10,000. Inside 42k, anything can happen.

It may well be that his best is yet to come.

The fastest men's marathons ever run

1	Dennis Kimetto (KEN)	Berlin	1st	28 September 2014	2:02:57

2	Geoffrey Mutai (KEN)	Boston	1st	18 April 2011	2:03:02
3	Eliud Kipchoge (KEN)	London	1st	24 April 2016	2:03:05
4	Moses Mosop (KEN)	Boston	2nd	18 April 2011	2:03:06
5	Emmanuel Mutai (KEN)	Berlin	2nd	28 September 2014	2:03:13
6	Wilson Kipsang (KEN)	Berlin	1st	29 September 2013	2:03:23
7	Patrick Makau (KEN)	Berlin	1st	25 September 2011	2:03:38
8	Wilson Kipsang (KEN)	Frankfurt	1st	30 October 2011	2:03:42
9	Stanley Biwott (KEN)	London	2nd	24 April 2016	2:03:51
10	Dennis Kimetto (KEN)	Chicago	1st	13 October 2013	2:03:45
11	Emmanuel Mutai (KEN)	Chicago	2nd	13 October 2013	2:03:52
12	Haile Gebrselassie (ETH)	Berlin	1st	28 September 2008	2:03:59

13	Eliud Kipchoge (KEN)	Berlin	1st	27 September 2015	2:04:00
14	Eliud Kipchoge (KEN)	Berlin	2nd	29 September 2013	2:04:05
15	Eliud Kipchoge (KEN)	Chicago	1st	12 October 2014	2:04:11
16	Geoffrey Mutai (KEN)	Berlin	1st	30 September 2012	2:04:15
17	Dennis Kimetto (KEN)	Berlin	2nd	30 September 2012	2:04:16
18	Ayele Absehero (ETH)	Dubai	1st	27 January 2012	2:04:23
19	Tesfaye Abera Dibaba (ETH)	Dubai	1st	22 January 2016	2:04:24
20	Haile Gebrselassie (ETH)	Berlin	1st	30 September 2007	2:04:26

Sammy Wanjiru – A tragic loss to marathon running

'He was one of our biggest heroes.
One of our best athletes ever.'
KENYAN MARATHON RUNNER
GODFREY KIPROTICH

In a career cut tragically short, Kenya's Sammy Wanjiru was – all too briefly – one of the brightest lights of men's marathon running, the winner of the overall World Marathon Majors title in 2009 and 2010.

Only 21 and already the holder of the world record in the half-marathon, Wanjiru (1986–2011) set a blistering pace from the off in the Beijing heat in the 2008 Olympic Games. Commentators doubted he could maintain it. But he did. Wanjiru was alone as he charged into the stadium at the end, shattering the Olympic record to finish in 2:06:32. It was Kenya's first gold medal in the Olympic marathon – and a massive highlight in Wanjiru's career.

As he told the *New York Times*:

> *I had to push the pace to tire the other runners. I had to push the pace because my body gets tired in the heat when I slow down. With 6 kilometres left, I tried to push. It was hard, but they didn't keep up.*

The following April, Wanjiru stormed to victory in the 2009 London Marathon, crossing the line in 2:05:10, 10 seconds ahead of Beijing bronze-medallist Tsegaye Kebede. Wanjiru had set out to break Haile Gebrselassie's world record, but the bid evaporated around the halfway mark. Even so, his time was a new London record.

As part of a remarkable run of marathon successes, Wanjiru followed up London by winning the Chicago Marathon later that year in a time of 2:05:41. He retained his Chicago title in 2010 with a time of 2:06:24, once again beating Ethiopian Tsegaye Kebede into second place, this time by 19 seconds.

Tragically, seven months later, Wanjiru was dead, after falling from a first-floor balcony at his home in the town of Nyahururu. Behind the tragedy was a history of marital problems. The December before, he had been charged with threatening to kill his wife, Triza Njeri – accusations she later withdrew. But his death came just days before he was due to appear in court on a firearms charge.

Many Kenyans believed his problems were linked to the fortune he had amassed from all his prize money and the adulation that surrounded him. There was certainly a great deal of soul-searching among other athletes. Had the athletics world done enough to help him cope with his success? Ethiopian great Gebrselassie tweeted a feeling many shared: 'One wonders if we as an athletics family could have avoided this tragedy.'

Former marathon world record holder Paul Tergat told the BBC:

> *We have lost a very young and talented athlete. This is a guy we were all hoping still had a long career ahead of him. He was only 24 years old so he still had about another ten years at the top of his career.*

National police spokesman Eric Kiraithe said Wanjiru killed himself but Nyahururu police chief Jasper Ombati said it may have been an accident. Wanjiru was pronounced dead in hospital after attempts to revive him failed. It seems likely the exact circumstances of his death will never been known.

His feats, however, will be long remembered. Virgin London Marathon race director Dave Bedford ranked him unquestionably the best:

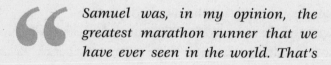

> *Samuel was, in my opinion, the greatest marathon runner that we have ever seen in the world. That's*

based on his amazing performance at the Olympics, but also the fact that he then went on to win two Chicago Marathons and one London Marathon. He was viewed by most people in the game as the person most likely to break Haile Gebrselassie's world record. He was a class athlete and a class human being.

Sammy Wanjiru's marathon record

10 October 2010	Chicago Marathon	2:06:23 (1st)
25 April 2010	London Marathon	did not finish
11 October 2009	Chicago Marathon	2:05:41 (1st)
26 April 2009	London Marathon	2:05:10 (1st)
24 August 2008	Beijing Olympic Marathon	2:06:32 (1st)
13 April 2008	London Marathon	2:05:24 (2nd)
2 December 2007	Fukuoka Marathon	2:06:39 (1st)

Dennis Kimetto – Chasing the 2-hour marathon

'I felt good from the start.'

On 28 September 2014, Kenyan Dennis Kimetto brought the time for the men's fastest marathon below 2 hours 3 minutes for the first time ever. His 2:02:57 was the sixth successive record to be set in Berlin.

Kimetto had promised to attack the record if conditions allowed, and he did so – a remarkable run from a 30-year-old who had started training seriously only four years before. Kimetto shook off the Kenyan Emmanuel Mutai with just under 3 miles to go. Mutai, who finished second in 2:03:13, also broke the previous record.

Kimetto said:

> *I feel good because I won a very tough race. I felt good from the start and in the last few miles I felt I could do it and break the record.*

Kimetto took the record from his friend and training partner Wilson Kipsang who set the previous standard with his time of 2:03:23 just a year before in Berlin. Dennis Kimetto, Wilson Kipsang and Emmanuel Mutai are the only three men who have twice run under the 2-hour 4-minute barrier. Kimetto acknowledged his debt to Kipsang in an interview in April 2015:

> *We are very committed together. It would be good to see us come in*

together. I love to run with him and working with him in training. He tells me to do this or that, go to speed work, a long run. He's taught me a lot. It is not just in this race. And he is my friend.

Born in 1984, Kimetto worked as a farmer, growing maize and looking after cows before joining Geoffrey Mutai's training group in 2008, and he finished second only to Geoffrey Mutai in Berlin in 2012. Kimetto's time was 2:04:16, the fastest debut marathon in history on a record-eligible course.

After his Berlin debut, Kimetto went on to win in Tokyo and Chicago in 2013; 2014 then saw his world record 2:02:57 (Berlin 2014), improving on his previous bests of 2:03:45 (Chicago 2013) and 2:04:16 (Berlin 2012) – results which stand respectively today as the first, eighth and fifteenth fastest times in marathon history. The consensus is that Kimetto, a late-starter in his chosen sport, brings to it a naturalness that stands him in great stead. Adharanand Finn, author of *Running with the Kenyans*, remarks:

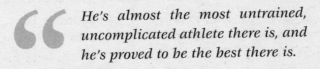

He's almost the most untrained, uncomplicated athlete there is, and he's proved to be the best there is.

Commenting on Kimetto's new record, Geoffrey Mutai saw it as confirmation that a 2-hour marathon is possible. Quite when that will happen, of course, nobody knows, but the race is certainly on.

In the meantime, despite the success, Kimetto has yet to give up farming. When he is not training, he also helps to build churches in his community and assists students with their school fees.

" *I also help young athletes who are at the start of their running career because they are now like I also used to be in the past and I know how important it is to be helped at the start. In the future they are the world record holders and champions so I find it important to help them.*

Men's marathon world record progression since 1980

26 April 1980	Gerard Nijboer (NED)	Amsterdam Marathon	2:09:01
6 December 1981	Robert de Castella (AUS)	Fukuoka Marathon	2:08:18
21 October 1984	Steve Jones (GBR)	Chicago Marathon	2:08:05
20 April 1985	Carlos Lopes (POR)	Rotterdam Marathon	2:07:12
17 April 1988	Belayneh Dinsamo (ETH)	Rotterdam Marathon	2:06:50
20 September 1998	Ronaldo da Costa (BRA)	Berlin Marathon	2:06:05
24 October 1999	Khalid Khannouchi (MOR)	Chicago Marathon	2:05:42

14 April 2002	Khalid Khannouchi (USA)	London Marathon	2:05:38
28 September 2003	Paul Tergat (KEN)	Berlin Marathon	2:04:55
30 September 2007	Haile Gebrselassie (ETH)	Berlin Marathon	2:04:26
28 September 2008	Haile Gebrselassie (ETH)	Berlin Marathon	2:03:59
25 September 2011	Patrick Makau (KEN)	Berlin Marathon	2:03:38
29 September 2013	Wilson Kipsang (KEN)	Berlin Marathon	2:03:23
28 September 2014	Dennis Kimetto (KEN)	Berlin Marathon	2:02:57

Mo Farah – 'It's great to make history'

*'I would say Mo is the greatest
sportsman Britain has ever had.'*
BRENDAN FOSTER, OLYMPIC MEDALLIST

Commentators and analysts struggle for superlatives when it
comes to Mo Farah, the first athlete to win three long-distance
doubles at successive world championships.

Farah's achievements are a far cry from his humble beginnings in
Somalia, arriving in London from Mogadishu at the age of eight

and speaking very little English. Growing up in West London, he began running at school. Spotted and encouraged by his PE teacher, Farah went on to become a very successful junior athlete winning the European Junior 5,000 m title in 2001. His major breakthrough on the senior stage came in 2006 when he won a silver medal in the 5,000 m in the European T&F Championships. An astonishing run of success has since given him national hero status in his adopted country.

In a world where perhaps too many champions are characterless automatons, Farah has character in abundance – one of the many reasons the country has taken him to its heart, in much the same way it got behind Paula Radcliffe in the early to mid-2000s.

Farah's website labels him 'the UK's greatest ever distance runner' – a claim richly justified by his status as double Olympic, European Athletics and World champion. As Paula Radcliffe observed: 'Mo is like a magician and he puts a spell over the whole field.'

In the Beijing Olympics in 2008, Farah failed to qualify for the 5,000 m final – a turning point. He vowed then to become the best in the world. The 2012 London Olympics were the best possible incentive.

The games arrived on a rising tide of expectation. Great Britain demanded that its athletes delivered, and they certainly did, with Farah leading the charge. On a golden night, in the same hour that Jessica Ennis won heptathlon gold and Greg Rutherford took the long jump gold, Farah buried his rivals with a blistering final lap to win the Olympic 10,000 m.

> *I just can't believe it. The crowd got so much behind me and was getting louder and louder. I've never experienced anything like this. It will never get any better than this. This is the best moment of my life.*

Farah was wrong. A week later, it did get better when he won the men's 5,000 m to claim his second Olympic gold. It was arguably the greater achievement. On season's bests, he was ranked only eleventh in the world at the start, but Farah took the lead at 600 m and finished the last 1,500 m in 4:00.5 to seal his victory. It was the moment he joined the sporting greats, the seventh man to win 5,000 m and 10,000 m gold at the same Olympics.

Farah went on to repeat the feat a year later, winning gold in both the 5,000 m and 10,000 m races at the 2013 World Championships.

The marathon was his next challenge and, inevitably, there was huge expectation when he made his debut in London in 2014. One of his hopes was to break the British marathon record of 2:07:13 set by Welshman Steve Jones when he won the Chicago Marathon in 1985. Sadly, it was not to be: Farah finished eighth in a time 2:08:21. Though naturally a huge disappointment to Farah and the watching public, it was nonetheless the fastest time by an Englishman, and the fourth fastest time by a Briton (Jones occupying the top three slots).

Despite the marathon disappointment, Farah continued to excel on the track and in August 2015, he made it six global distance titles in a row. Following on from his Olympic double in the 2012 and his double at the 2013 World Championships, he achieved the double again in the 2015 World Championships in Beijing. The 10,000 m gold came hand in hand with the 5,000 m gold once again, and history was made. Mo Farah became the first man ever to achieve a distance 'triple double'.

Olympic medallist and now commentator Brendan Foster was unstinting in his praise:

Tonight has put him at the top table. When you talk about the greatest distance runners of the world,

he has gone alongside them. He is up there with the greats, Haile Gebrselassie, Kenenisa Bekele, Emil Zátopek and Lasse Virén. [...] This guy is still adding to his record books. He is getting better as he gets older.

Career highlights

2015 IAAF World T&F Championships, 5,000 m and 10,000 m	Gold
2015 European Half-marathon	Record
2014 New York Half-marathon	2nd
2014 London Marathon	8th
2014 Great North Run Half-marathon	1st
2014 Diamond League Birmingham, 2 miles	1st
2014 European Championships Zurich, 5,000 m	1st
2014 European Championships Zurich, 10,000 m	1st
2013 New Orleans Half-marathon	1st
2013 World Championships, 10,000 m	Gold
2013 World Championships, 5,000 m	Gold

2012 Olympic Games London, 10,000 m	Gold
2012 Olympic Games London, 5,000 m	Gold
2011 World Championships, 5,000 m	Gold
2011 World Championships, 10,000 m	Silver
2011 New York Half-marathon	1st
2011 European Indoor, 3,000 m	Gold
2010 European T&F Championships, 5,000 m	Gold
2010 European T&F Championships, 10,000 m	Gold

CHAPTER FOURTEEN

THE MOST EXTRAORDINARY RUN OF ALL

Tim Peake – Out of this world!

'This morning was fantastic.'

Some runs might be described as out of this world, but Tim Peake's 2016 'London Marathon' literally was.

As tens of thousands of runners completed 26.2 miles around the streets of London, astronaut Tim Peake gave new meaning to the term 'runner's high' when he ran an identical distance hundreds of miles above the earth.

The first Briton to be selected by the European Space Agency (ESA) for a mission to the International Space Station, Peake provided the countdown for the thirty-sixth London Marathon before running his own virtual version of the race. A recorded message, in which Peake wished the competitors good luck, was played on big screens before the runners set off in London. But, while his earthbound counterparts increasingly felt the weight of their wearying bodies, Peake was strapped to a treadmill to counter the lack of gravity in the International Space Station – a fact that presented its own set of difficulties, as he explained:

> *One of the biggest challenges is the harness system. Obviously, my body-weight has to be firmly attached to the treadmill by this harness, and that can rub on the shoulders and around the waist.*

Dressed in a red vest and black shorts, 44-year-old Peake was somewhere over the Pacific Ocean when he started. By the time he had finished, he had travelled more than twice around the planet. In effect, while the London runners covered 26.2 miles, Peake – with a little space station assistance – covered 53,000 miles during his run.

Behind him every step of the way was the Union Flag. While the runners down below grabbed at their drinks from the water stations along the way, Peake's water pouch was velcroed to the wall above his head. While the terrestrial marathoners had the sights of the capital to spur them on, Peake was in a windowless room, reliant on technology to keep his spirits up.

Peake later blogged:

> *Watching the live marathon on the BBC the whole time was a huge encouragement – I had thought I*

would watch a movie (2001: A Space Odyssey was ready to go) or listen to my #Spacerocks playlist but in fact it was extremely motivating watching the live coverage of the event and hearing the stories of some of the 33,000 people taking part. In addition to that I was able to compare my progress to the live event since I had the RunSocial app giving me an excellent view of streets of London as I would see them if I were running the real marathon.

Peake's achievement was a remarkable one, and one in defiance of the weakening effects of weightlessness during his months in space. Daily exercise is essential for astronauts as they fight to prevent their aerobic fitness and muscle strength from fading. Although Peake had completed the London Marathon in 1999 in 3 hours, 18 minutes and 50 seconds, in space he was advised against trying to beat his time to ensure he was in good shape for his return to earth two months later, in June. He finished his virtual marathon in 3 hours, 35 minutes and 21 seconds.

Peake, who was running to raise awareness of The Prince's Trust, was not the first astronaut to run a marathon in space. NASA astronaut Sunita Williams ran alongside the Boston Marathon in 2007, finishing in 4 hours and 24 minutes. Experts point out the two runs cannot be compared, as the two astronauts ran with different harnesses and different loads. But Peake's quicker run was more than enough for Marco Frigatti, from the Guinness World Records. He confirmed: 'It's official. Tim Peake is the proud holder of a Guinness World Record title.'

REFERENCES

CHAPTER ONE:
RUNNING FINDS ITS FEET

PHEIDIPPIDES
Herodotus, *The Histories*, VI

DEERFOOT
www.sni.org, website of the Seneca Nation of Indians
Edward S. Sears, *Running through the Ages* (2001)
New York Times, 20 January 1896

CHARLES ROWELL
New Zealand Herald, 16 October 1909
Ottawa Citizen, 16 October 1909

DORANDO PIETRI
New York Times, 25 July 1908

ARTHUR NEWTON
Oxford Dictionary of National Biography
www.sabc.co.za/news/a/fabed6004b721acd8170ad78893a5284/
  Comrades-runners-advised-to-honour-halfway-mark-
  tradition-20123105
www.comrades.com
John Cameron-Dow, *Comrades Marathon: The Ultimate Human Race*,
  (2011)

PAAVO NURMI

Cordner Nelson, *Track's Greatest Champions* (1986)
Guardian, 1925
Gabriel Hanot, *Le Miroir des Sports*, 1924

ROGER BANNISTER

www.theguardian.com/uk-news/2015/sep/11/roger-bannisters-
sub-four-minute-mile-running-shoes-sell-for-266500
www.telegraph.co.uk/sport/othersports/athletics/10803219/I-
gave-it-everything-Sir-Roger-Bannister-marks-60-years-since-his-
record.html

CHAPTER TWO:
TRULY INSPIRATIONAL

JANE TOMLINSON

www.theguardian.com/theobserver/2004/may/16/features.review7
www.janetomlinsonappeal.com
www.dailymail.co.uk/femail/article-2260692/Jane-Tomlinsons-
husband-inspiring-legacy-continues-launch-Yorkshire-Marathon.
html

HYVON NGETICH

www.fox7austin.com/news/614153-story
www.huffingtonpost.com/2015/02/17/hyvon-ngetich-crawls-
finish-line-austin-marathon-2015_n_6697488.html
www.foxsports.com.au/news/hyvon-ngetich-crawls-on-hands-and-
knees-to-cross-finish-line-in-inspirational-performance/news-story/5f
55522ccccc710ec138e14cca49f333
edition.cnn.com/2015/02/16/us/austin-marathon-finish-line-crawl/

EDDIE IZZARD

www.theguardian.com/culture/2009/sep/15/eddie-izzard-charity-
run
www.telegraph.co.uk/tv/2016/03/18/sport-relief-2016-live-eddie-
izzard-luthers-idris-elba-and-jo-br/
Reader's Digest, May 2013
www.bbc.co.uk/news/entertainment-arts-35856814

TERRY FOX

www.terryfox.org

BRUCE CLELAND

www.spryliving.com/articles/team-in-training-the-little-girl-who-
started-a-running-revolution-video
www.running.competitor.com/2013/01/features/bruce-cleland-
the-first-charity-runner_65166

JENNIFER SHERIDAN

www.begoodbestrong.blogspot.co.uk
archive.boston.com/yourtown/boston/fenway_kenmore/
articles/2012/04/15/marbleheads_jennifer_sheridan_puts_her_
heart_into_marathon_run/

CHAPTER THREE: THE PIONEERS
OF WOMEN'S DISTANCE RUNNING

VIOLET PIERCY

www.nuts.org.uk/trackstats/piercy.htm
www.oxforddnb.com/index/103/101103698/
www.britishpathe.com/video/camera-interviews-the-runner

DALE GREIG

www.independent.co.uk/sport/the-winners-who-werent-trail-blazer-who-broke-the-rules-1234101.html

www.heraldscotland.com/sport/13211016.Take_a_bow_Paula__but_you_owe_it_all_to_Dale

BOBBI GIBB

www.nytlive.nytimes.com/womenintheworld/2015/04/20/the-incredible-story-of-bobbi-gibb-the-first-woman-to-run-the-boston-marathon

www.audio.californiareport.org/archive/R201304150850/b

www.eatrunread.com/2012/04/bobbi-gibb-first-woman-to-run-boston.html

KATHRINE SWITZER

Kathrine Switzer, *Marathon Woman* (2009)

www.boston.com/sports/boston-marathon/2015/04/18/kathrine-switzer-on-the-marathon-moment-that-changed-millions-of-womens-lives

CHAPTER FOUR:
BECAUSE IT'S THERE

DAVE MCGILLIVRAY

www.bostonglobe.com/lifestyle/style/2014/03/20/dave-mcgillivray-marathon-transformedLe74Cv04u34yBTdqLFJkyO/story.html

www.running.competitor.com/2015/04/boston-marathon/dave-did-it-again-mcgillivray-finishes-43rd-straight-boston-marathon_126934

AMY HUGHES

www.bbc.co.uk/news/uk-england-shropshire-29359358
www.telegraph.co.uk/news/uknews/11125322/Young-womans-incredible-achievement-of-53-marathons-in-53-days.html
www.53marathons.co.uk
www.shropshirestar.com/news/2015/04/08/stepping-out-shropshire-marathon-star-amy-hughes-runs-into-the-arms-of-love

KIM ALLAN

www.nydailynews.com/news/world/new-zealand-woman-breaks-record-running-sleep-article-1.1556206
http://www.stuff.co.nz/auckland/local-news/local-blogs/running-auckland/9611455/An-Interview-with-Ultra-Runner-Kim-Allan
www.telegraph.co.uk/news/worldnews/australiaandthepacific/newzealand/10533677/Woman-breaks-the-record-for-running-without-sleep.html
www.nzherald.co.nz/nz/news/article.cfm?c_id=1&object id=11176746.

ACHIM ARETZ

www.npr.org/2012/03/11/148398083/record-setter-says-he-wont-run-backward-anymore
Backwards Running (1981)

FIONA OAKES

www.vivalavegan.net/interviews/3-articles/294-interview-with-fiona-oakes-vegan-marathon-runner.html
www.greatveganathletes.com
www.towerhillstables.com

JON SUTHERLAND

www.espn.go.com/sports/endurance/story/_/id/9834548/
endurance-sports-44-years-jon-sutherland-running-streak-going-
strong

www.latimes.com/sports/highschool/lat-sp-jon-sutherland-1-
20140525-photo.html

The Official USA Active Running Streak List

RICK WORLEY

www.washingtonpost.com/wp-dyn/articles/A407-2004Oct26.html

www.prnewswire.com/news-releases/world-record-marathoner-to-
end-consecutive-running-streak-71979132.html

DAVID AND LINDA MAJOR

www.madeyarun.com

JEN CORREA

www.momsgottarun.com

www.experiencelife.com/article/after-the-storm-jen-correas-
success-story

www.everymothercounts.org

www.edition.cnn.com/2012/11/02/us/sandy-nyc-marathon

CHAPTER FIVE: THE LEGENDS OF MEN'S DISTANCE RUNNING

EMIL ZÁTOPEK

New York Herald Tribune 1952

www.theguardian.com/sport/blog/2012/jun/22/50-olympic-stunning-
moments-emil-zatopek

edition.cnn.com/2012/08/11/sport/london-olympics-zatopek-
marathon

www.nytimes.com/2000/11/23/sports/emil-zatopek-78-ungainly-
running-star-dies.html

JIM PETERS
www.theguardian.com/sport/2007/jan/07/athletics.features

KIP KEINO
www.bristol.ac.uk/pace/graduation/honorary-degrees/hondeg07/
  keino.html
www.kipkeinofoundation.co.ke

STEVE PREFONTAINE
www.running.competitor.com/2015/05/photos/14-great-steve-
  prefontaine-quotes_127591
USA Track & Field, www.usatf.org
www.runnersworld.com/runners-stories/why-pre-still-matters

CHRIS BRASHER
www.britishathletics.org.uk/e-inspire/hall-of-fame-athletes/chris-
  brasher
www.theguardian.com/news/2003/mar/01/guardianobituaries
www.dailymail.co.uk/columnists/article-301526/Farewell-Chris-
  gave-gold-fighting-spirit.html

HAILE GEBRSELASSIE
www.bbc.co.uk/sport/athletics/32680723

PAUL TERGAT
www.takethemagicstep.com/inspiration/interviews/paul-tergat-
  passion-determination-and-belief-lead-to-success
www.paultergat-foundation.org

CHAPTER SIX:
DEFEATING THE TERRORISTS

THERESA GIAMMONA
www.crowdrise.com/nypoliceandfireNYC2015/fundraiser/
  theresagiammona
www.runnersworld.com/new-york-city-marathon/for-widow-of-
  firefighter-who-died-on-september-11-the-race-is-finally-run

KEVIN PARKS
www.huffingtonpost.com/2013/09/11/kevin-parks-9-11-boston-
  marathon_n_3906667.html

BRIAN KELLEY
www.whitehouse.gov/the-press-office/2013/04/18/remarks-
  president-interfaith-service-boston-ma
www.pavementrunner.com
www.runrocknroll.com

JULI WINDSOR
www.juliwindsor.com
www.today.com/news/year-its-so-much-more-runners-dwarfism-
  make-inspiring-return-2D79467846
www.bostonglobe.com/metro/2013/04/30/first-dwarfs-run-boston-
  marathon-finish-route/70JHV4bZ8DIgv9oiFO4pqL/story.html
www.artery.wbur.org/2014/12/23/boston-marathon-abel-windsor-
  documentary

LYNN CRISCI
www.uspainfoundation.org
www.facebook.com/PopSuperhero

GEORGES SALINES

www.lemonde.fr/attaques-a-paris/visuel/2015/12/10/lola-salines-29-ans-enmemoire_4829310_4809495.html

www.20minutes.fr/societe/1814107-20160326-attaques-terroristes-paris-reconstruction-marathon-georges-salines

CHAPTER SEVEN:
CONQUERING DISABILITY

DAVID KUHN

www.itsallicando.wordpress.com

www.bismarcktribune.com/news/state-and-regional/blind-man-running-for-granddaughter/article_8e5ad126-121d-11e4-b789-001a4bcf887a.html

www.runhaven.com/2014/07/10/forrest-gump-nothing-david-kuhn

TEAM HOYT

www.teamhoyt.com/About-Team-Hoyt.html

www.bostonglobe.com/sports/2014/04/22/dick-and-rick-hoyt-run-marathon-their-last-duo/0802xdlCGKe5Z84VmCgMpI/story.html

www.abcnews.go.com/Health/team-hoyt-run-boston-marathon/story?id=23288967

THE SCHNEIDER TWINS

www.autismrunners.com

www.nytimes.com/2013/05/05/sports/autistic-twins-find-a-release-in-running.html?_r=0

www.espn.go.com/sports/endurance/story/_/id/12703126/endurance-sports-autistic-twins-alex-jamie-schneider-bring-inspiration-boston-marathon

CLAIRE LOMAS

www.bbc.co.uk/news/uk-england-leicestershire-17988848

www.spinalresearch.org

www.mirror.co.uk/news/real-life-stories/claire-lomas-inspiring-story-life-1879107

www.claireschallenge.co.uk

MAICKEL MELAMED

www.dailymail.co.uk/news/article-3048840/Venezuelan-man-finish-Boston-Marathon-20-hours.html

www.masslive.com/news/boston/index.ssf/2015/04/boston_marathon_2015_maickel_m.html

www.boston.cbslocal.com/2015/04/21/boston-marathons-final-finisher-an-inspirational-story/

www.maickelmelamed.com

PHIL PACKER

www.telegraph.co.uk/sport/olympics/paralympic-sport/5304281/Major-Phil-Packer-completes-London-Marathon.html

www.britishinspirationtrust.org.uk

CHAPTER EIGHT: THE 80s GREATS OF WOMEN'S DISTANCE RUNNING

GRETE WAITZ

www.nytimes.com/2011/04/20/sports/othersports/20waitz.html

INGRID KRISTIANSEN

www.nydailynews.com/sports/more-sports/marathon-organizers-deny-conpiracty-ensure-waitz-success-article-1.1500059

www.si.com/vault/1986/10/27/114242/the-best-norse-in-the-long-run-ingrid-kristiansen-of-norway-a-skier-turned-runner-is-the-fastest-woman-in-the-world-over-5000-meters-10000-meters--and-in-the-marathon
www.iaaf.org/athletes/norway/ingrid-kristiansen-61007#personal-bests

ROSA MOTA
www.youtube.com/watch?v=8NudILf8jJ0
www.time-to-run.com/marathon/athletes/women/mota

JOAN BENOIT SAMUELSON
www.nyrr.org/about-us/nyrr-hall-of-fame/joan-benoit-samuelson
www.running.competitor.com

CHAPTER NINE:
WHEN THE MIND IS WILLING

KIM STEMPLE
www.phxux.krem.com/story/news/local/dc/2015/10/23/dc-marathoner-collecting-medals-inspire-sick/74487354
www.runnersworld.com/runners-stories/woman-with-terminal-illness-runs-her-last-marathon
www.wefinishtogether.com

PATRICK FINNEY
www.reuters.com/article/us-multiple-sclerosis-marathon-idUSTRE78P4HN20110926
www.sportsday.dallasnews.com/other-sports/runningheadlines/2011/09/22/fetterman-grapevine-runner-set-to-become-first-individual-with-ms-to-complete-marathon-in-all-50-states
www.marathonmaniacsdb.com/Maniacs/MyRaces/2149

ELIZABETH MAIUOLO

www.womenshealthmag.com/fitness/running-inspiration-heart-
attack-survivor-tackles-the-marathon

www.runningandthecity.com

MICHAEL LAFORGIA

www.nmaus.org/stories/nma-advocates/new-york

www.runnersworld.com/new-york-city-marathon/inspiring-
runners-of-the-new-york-city-marathon

www.lipulse.com/2015/08/31/silver-linings

DON WRIGHT

www.patientsrising.org

www.businesswire.com/news/home/20151124005249/en/Patients-
Rising-Honors-Cancer-Patient-Don-Wright

wtop.com/local/2015/10/cancer-fight-fuels-runners-marathon-
feats/slide/1

MARK MCGIRR

www.running.competitor.com/2015/10/rock-n-roll-marathon-
series/a-second-life-runner-returns-to-rock-n-roll-vancouver-
with-doctor-who-saved-him_138214

www.cbc.ca/news/canada/british-columbia/heart-attack-victim-
runs-with-doctor-who-saved-his-life-1.3286979

CHAPTER TEN: PUSHING THE LIMITS OF HUMAN ENDURANCE

TED JACKSON
www.overcomingms.org
www.dailymail.co.uk/femail/article-2956995/Husband-runs-
seven-marathons-world-SEVEN-days-raises-160K-multiple-
sclerosis-childhood-sweetheart-diagnosed.html
www.independent.co.uk/news/people/the-man-set-to-run-seven-
marathons-on-seven-continents-in-seven-days-to-raise-money-
for-ms-charity-9946601.html
www.iknowtedjackson.com

ANGELA TORTORICE
www.espn.go.com/espnw/journeys-victories/article/8111766/
espnw-angela-tortorice-maniacally-devoted-marathons
www.dmagazine.com/publications/d-magazine/2012/february/
marathon-woman-angela-tortorice

DEAN KARNAZES
Dean Karnazes, *Ultramarathon Man: Confessions of an All-Night Runner*
(2006)
www.theguardian.com/lifeandstyle/the-running-blog/2013/
aug/30/dean-karnazes-man-run-forever

STEFAAN ENGELS
www.content.time.com/time/health/article/0,8599,2048604,00.html
www.marathonman365movie.be

ROB YOUNG
www.skysports.com/more-sports/athletics/news/29877/
9883585/marathon-man-rob-young-aims-for-record-breaking-summer
www.marathonmanuk.com
www.telegraph.co.uk/men/active/11561584/My-childhood-abuse-
spurred-me-on-to-run-370-marathons-in-a-year.html

KEVIN CARR

www.hardwayround.com

www.telegraph.co.uk/men/active/11524386/Meet-the-British-ultra-runner-whos-set-to-complete-a-remarkable-world-record.html

www.dailymail.co.uk/news/article-3032867/I-ve-British-athlete-fastest-man-run-round-world-621-days-despite-attacked-bears-hunted-wolves-run-TWICE.html

www.bbc.co.uk/news/uk-england-devon-32195535

www.sane.org.uk/how_you_can_help/blogging/show_blog/645

PAUL STASO

www.coolrunning.com/engine/6/6_1/montana-man-runs-across-a.shtml

www.paulstaso.com

CLIFF YOUNG

www.elitefeet.com/the-legend-of-Cliff-Young

www.smh.com.au/articles/2003/11/03/1067708126175.html

MARATHON MANIAC LARRY

www.runnersworld.com/newswire/69-year-old-breaks-record-for-most-marathons-in-a-year

www.ksat.com/news/local-runner-70-finishes-1410th-marathon

espn.go.com/sports/endurance/story/_/id/10289954/endurance-sports-record-marathoner-larry-macon-slowing-down

www.ksat.com/news/self-proclaimed-marathon-maniac-runs-again

www.mysanantonio.com/news/news_columnists/jan_jarboe_russell/article/What-makes-Larry-Macon-run-972646.php

ISTVAN SIPOS

www.srichinmoy.org

www.nytimes.com/1994/08/21/sports/ultramarathon-2926-miles-in-517-hours-wins-race.html

JC SANTA TERESA

www.rocklandroadrunners.org/2015/02/jc-santa-teresa-sets
  guinness-world-record
www.lohud.com/story/news/local/rockland/2015/06/26
  ultramarathoner-hits-two-hundred/29354635

CHAPTER ELEVEN:
IN THE TOUGHEST PLACES

MAURO PROSPERI

www.marathondessables.co.uk
www.bbc.co.uk/news/magazine-30046426

DAVE HEELEY

www.marathondessables.co.uk
www.britishblindsport.org.uk
www.birminghammail.co.uk/news/midlands-news/blind-dave-
  heeley-wins-award-7573933
www.blinddaveheeley.co.uk

ENGLE, ZAHAB AND LIN

www.washingtonpost.com/wp-dyn/content/article/2007/
  02/20/AR2007022000856_pf.html
www.runningthesahara.com
water.org

SCOTT JUREK

www.nytimes.com/2010/05/13/sports/13runner.html
www.spartathlon.gr
www.impactmagazine.ca/features/35-feature-articles/252-
  interview-with-scott-jurek
www.nomeatathlete.com

PAT FARMER

www.timesofisrael.com/a-forrest-gump-run-for-peace
www.gadling.com/2013/06/21/meet-pat-farmer-the-aussie-who-ran-20-919-kilometers-from-pole
www.redcross.org.au

SCOTT AND RHYS JENKINS

www.badwater.com
www.operationsmile.org.uk
www.walesonline.co.uk

SIR RANULPH FIENNES

www.news.bbc.co.uk/1/hi/world/americas/3234479.stm
www.mariecurie.org.uk

NICHOLAS BOURNE

www.news.bbc.co.uk/1/hi/world/africa/228660.stm
www.gomulti.co.za/tag/nicholas-bourne

MALCOLM ATTARD

www.timesofmalta.com/articles/view/20131228/athletics/Maltese-endurance-runner-beats-Mount-Everest-race-challenge.500526
www.timesofmalta.com/articles/view/20120602/local/Athlete-to-tackle-gruelling-ultra-marathon-for-charity.422353
www.everestmarathon.org.uk

CHAPTER TWELVE:
AGE SHALL NOT WEARY...

FAUJA SINGH

www.guinnessworldrecords.com/news/2011/10/statement-from-guinness-world-records-fauja-singh

www.bbc.co.uk/news/world-us-canada-15330421

www.theguardian.com/lifeandstyle/the-running-blog/2013/oct/11/fauja-singh-worlds-oldest-runner-102

BOB DOLPHIN

www.seattletimes.com/sports/other-sports/running-bob-dolphin-80-is-no-run-of-the-mill-marathoner

JOY JOHNSON

www.nytimes.com/news/the-lives-they-lived/2013/12/21/joy-johnson/

www.nyrr.org

www.today.com/news/famed-runner-joy-johnson-86-dies-one-day-after-nyc-8C11535662

ESPN's 30-for-30 series of short films

www.facebook.com/inmemoryJoyJohnson

LOUISE ROSSETTI

www.bostonglobe.com/metro/2014/07/06/louise-rossetti-saugus-inspirational-runner-competed-thousands-races-into-her-late/yhsaK9zHvrUHqY9xhhQM8J/story.html

www.saugus.wickedlocal.com/article/20140716/News/140717743

SISTER MADONNA BUDER

www.dailymail.co.uk/femail/article-2617187/I-just-boogie-Meet-82-year-old-Iron-Nun-completed-340-triathlons-one-month-30-years.html

www.cosmopolitan.com/health-fitness/advice/a6538/iron-nun-sister-madonna-buder-triathlon-ironman-and-marathon-runner/

SAB KOIDE

well.blogs.nytimes.com/2009/09/02/inspiration-for-runners-over-50/

www.nyrr.org/races-and-events/2012/race-to-deliver/race-recap

GLADYS BURRILL AND HARRIETTE THOMPSON

www.dailymail.co.uk/news/article-1373513/Meet-Gladys-ator-Woman-92-breaks-world-record-finishes-marathon.html

www.nbcnews.com/id/42427918/ns/us_news-life/t/-year-old-marathoners-secret-think-positive/#.Vob2hqunWiY

www.news.adventist.org

www.foxnews.com/us/2015/05/31/2-year-old-becomes-oldest-woman-to-finish-marathon.html

www.charlotteobserver.com/news/local/article22753806.html

CHAPTER THIRTEEN:
THE MODERN GREATS

CATHERINE NDEREBA

www.old.post-gazette.com/sports/other/20020507kenya0507p3.asp

www.articles.chicagotribune.com/2002-10-10/sports/0210100353_1_jane-catherine-ndereba-trains

TEGLA LOROUPE

www.wsj.com/articles/SB100014240527023038431045791698815 99887664

www.biographyonline.net/sport/tegla-loroupe.html

www.nytimes.com/2006/11/18/world/africa/18tegla.html?ref=topics&_r=0

PAULA RADCLIFFE

www.theguardian.com/sport/2013/apr/20/paula-radcliffe-london-marathon-record

www.news.bbc.co.uk/sport1/hi/athletics/london_marathon_2003/2945709.stm

www.bbc.co.uk/sport/athletics/22184970

www.bbc.co.uk/sport/athletics/32473497

MARY KEITANY

www.tcsnycmarathon.org

www.bbc.co.uk/sport/athletics/17803863

www.iaaf.org

GEOFFREY MUTAI

www.takethemagicstep.com/news-events/sports-stories/geoffrey-mutai-runs-worlds-best-at-the-boston-marathon/

KENENISA BEKELE

www.iaaf.org

www.running.competitor.com/2015/01/news/kenenisa-bekele-bringing-new-weapon-dubai-experience_121466

SAMMY WANJIRU

www.telegraph.co.uk/sport/olympics/8516077/London-2012-Olympics-Sammy-Wanjiru-the-best-male-marathon-runner-ever-says-David-Bedford.html

www.theguardian.com/world/2011/may/16/olympic-athlete-death-kenya-wanjiru

DENNIS KIMETTO
www.bbc.co.uk/sport/athletics/29399623
www.channel4.com/news/dennis-kimetto-marathon-running-kenya-how
www.independent.co.uk/sport/general/athletics/london-marathon-2015-kenyas-brothers-in-arms-wilson-kipsang-and-dennis-kimetto-ready-to-take-on-10200083.html
www.sub2hrs.com

MO FARAH
www.mofarah.com
www.bbc.co.uk/sport/olympics/18912882
www.bbc.co.uk/sport/athletics/34092438

CHAPTER FOURTEEN: THE MOST EXTRAORDINARY RUN OF ALL

TIM PEAKE
www.theguardian.com/science/2016/apr/24/runners-high-tim-peake-finishes-london-marathon-in-space
www.bbc.co.uk/news/science-environment-36112137
www.telegraph.co.uk/news/2016/04/24/watch-live-tim-peake-runs-the-london-marathon-on-the-internation/
www.blogs.esa.int/tim-peake/2016/04/25/marathon-run/
www.virginmoneylondonmarathon.com/en-gb/news-media/latest-news/item/astronaut-to-run-virgin-money-london-marathon-in-space/

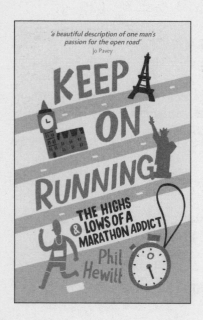

KEEP ON RUNNING

Phil Hewitt

ISBN: 978 1 84953 236 5

Paperback

£8.99

Marathons make you miserable, but they also give you the most unlikely and the most indescribable pleasures. It's a world that I love – a world unlocked when you dress up in lycra, put plasters on your nipples and run 26.2 miles in the company of upwards of 30,000 complete strangers.

Phil Hewitt, who has completed 30 marathons in conditions ranging from blistering heat to snow and ice, in locations round the globe from London to New York, sets a cracking pace in this story of an ordinary guy's addiction to marathon running. Reliving the highs and lows along the way, this light-hearted account of his adventures on the road examines the motivation that keeps you going when your body is crying out to stop. Above all, it tries to answer the ultimate question: 'Why do you do it?'

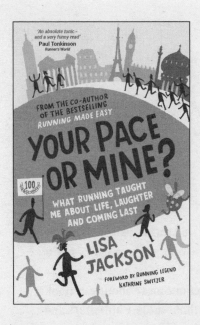

YOUR PACE OR MINE?

Lisa Jackson

ISBN: 978 1 84953 827 5

Paperback

£9.99

Lisa Jackson is a surprising cheerleader for the joys of running. Formerly a committed fitness-phobe, she became a marathon runner at 31, and ran her first 56-mile ultramarathon aged 41. And unlike many runners, Lisa's not afraid to finish last – in fact, she's done so in 20 of the 90-plus marathons she's completed so far.

But this isn't just Lisa's story, it's also that of the extraordinary people she's met along the way – tutu-clad fun-runners, octogenarians and 250-mile ultrarunners – whose tales of loss and laughter are sure to inspire you just as much as they've inspired her. This book is for anyone who longs to experience the sense of connection and achievement that running has to offer, whether a nervous novice or a seasoned marathoner dreaming of doing an ultra. An account of the triumph of tenacity over a lack of talent, *Your Pace or Mine?* is proof that running really isn't about the time you do, but the time you have!

Have you enjoyed this book?
If so, why not write a review on your favourite website?

If you're interested in finding out more about our books,
find us on Facebook at **Summersdale Publishers** and
follow us on Twitter at **@Summersdale**.

Thanks very much for buying this Summersdale book.

www.summersdale.com